Heal Your Pelvic Floor, LIVE YOUR LIFE!

Part V of the "Live Your Life!" Series

By: Dr. Sara S. Morrison

In loving memory of Richard Carl Morrison.
You were the best Father-in-Law
anyone could ever ask for.
Thank you for always loving me like one of
your own, Dad!

We will hold you in our Hearts,
Until we can hold you in Heaven.

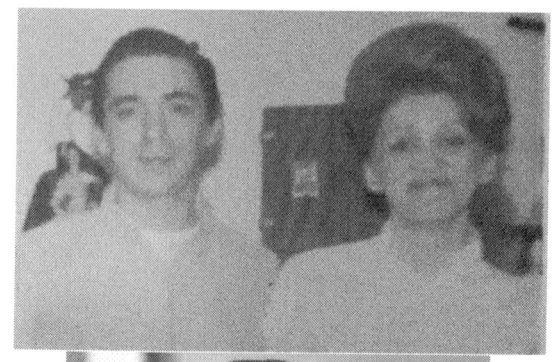

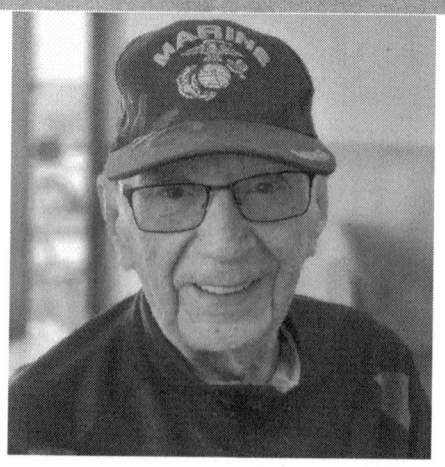

November 9, 1936 — June 12, 2021

Special Thank You to:

My Editor, Vicky Grady

Without you, the number of grammar mistakes would be immeasurable!
Thank you from the bottom of my heart for all your time and talents!

And

My Amazing Book Chapter Models!

Blake Patrick Morrison
Erik Morrison
Sue Muto
Linda Muto
Marlene Snyder
Tricia Buchheit
Caroline Buchheit
Gianna Smith
(What a beautiful and talented family I have!)

Table of Contents

Introduction	6
Chapter 1: My Pelvic Floor Story	11
Chapter 2: What is the Pelvic Floor?	17
Chapter 3: What Causes the Pelvic Floor Not to Work Correctly?	20
Chapter 4: What Does Pelvic Floor Dysfunction Feel Like?	26
Chapter 5: Pelvic Floor Dysfunction in Men	29
Chapter 6: Pelvic Floor Dysfunction in Women	47
Chapter 7: Other Factors That Increase Pelvic Floor Dysfunction	53
Chapter 8: Incontinence Myths	60
Chapter 9: Types of Incontinence	64
Chapter 10: Pelvic Organ Prolapse	69
Chapter 11: Diastasis Recti (Six-Pack Abs)	78
Chapter 12: How Do I Fix My Pelvic Floor?	84
Chapter 13: Breathing Pattern	88
Chapter 14: 360-Degree Breathing Pattern	96
Chapter 15: Pressure	100
Chapter 16: What Does Bad Breathing Do?	109
Chapter 17: All Conversations Lead to Posture	117
Chapter 18: Kegels	127
Chapter 19: Putting It All Together	135

Chapter 20: Top Ten Common Pelvic Floor Questions	145
Chapter 21: Exercises – Simple Ways to Fix Your Pelvic Floor	159
Patient Testimonials	169
References	185
About the Author	189
SPECIAL OFFER - Free Wellness Check-Up & Deep Tissue Laser Consultation	191

INTRODUCTION:

Do you leak when you cough, laugh, or sneeze?

When you have the urge to go to the bathroom, do you "Have to go RIGHT NOW?"

Do you have erectile dysfunction?

Do you have pain with intercourse or using a tampon?

Do you have trouble fully emptying your bowel or bladder?

Do you feel weak or "broken" after having a baby?

Have you been told you have prolapse, or had prostate surgery?

Are you tired of missing activities with family and loved ones because of your leaking?

No one likes to talk about leaking, not even with their doctor. Many people think leaking is normal after having a baby, abdominal pelvic surgery, or getting older. THAT'S WRONG! Leaking is "common" after these issues, but it is NOT normal, and there are things you can do to correct it. Things that do NOT involve medication, injections, or surgery.

Over the years, I have found it increasingly hard for people to find accurate information on healing their bodies naturally. Sure, there is a ton of information out there! But search "pelvic floor" or "leaking" on the internet, and thousands upon thousands of sites will come up. But is it accurate? Can you really believe it?

Most people are too embarrassed or ashamed to talk about leaking, prolapse, ED, or other concerns, even with their doctor. So how are they supposed to find accurate information on improving these issues? I wrote this book to let people know that you do not have to live with these problems. I hope you find it informative. Please feel free to share it with a friend. You never know which of your loved ones is one of the millions of people silently suffering from Pelvic Floor Dysfunction.

If you don't know me, here's how I started on the path that led me to Harnett County and Total Body Therapy & Wellness.

I graduated from PT school in 2002 and I headed South. I always wanted to live in the sunshine by the beach. The plan was for my husband (fiancé at the time) and I to move to Virginia Beach for about 2 years, get some experience, and then move back to Western New York. I was going to get a job at the local hospital, have my 2.5 kids, and lead a quiet life.

However, that was not God's plan for me.

We changed plans to target North Carolina. As I continued looking for jobs, I found myself falling in love with North Carolina. I had one interview there. It was a horrible job, but I LOVED the area! One hot summer day, I found myself in Harnett County in a small waiting room. I was a 21-year-old girl, far away from home, nervous and sweating in my heavy black suit. As I was waiting for my interview, several of the patients in the waiting room began talking to me. They were so friendly and genuine. They eased my nerves and helped me relax. When I walked off to my interview, they even hugged me and wished me good luck! Something told me I had just found my new home... and the interview had not even begun! It turns out my husband had a very similar experience talking to people at the gas station as he waited for me. We both knew Harnett County was where we belonged! As time went on, we continued to fall in love with North Carolina, the people, the strong family values... and of course... the sun!

Several years after living in North Carolina I lost my job. I literally walked up to find the Sheriff locking the door.

"Don't bother," he said, "This place is closed." I came home sad and afraid. We were barely making ends meet as it was.

What about my patients? Where would they go? I knew they would not travel to Raleigh or Fayetteville for care. Most people would just go on hurting. I did not want that to happen.

It was then that my husband convinced me to open my own clinic. He helped me remember my frustrations about not being able to treat my patients the way I wanted. This would give me the opportunity to do that! With his unending support and encouragement, I opened Total Body Therapy & Wellness in July of 2008. My plan was to operate this by myself for 6 months or a year. By then I would hopefully have enough money to hire an office person. My long-term goal, in my wildest dreams, was that I would one day have enough need for a rehab technician, an office person, and maybe, just maybe, a PT Assistant.

Yet again, the Big Man upstairs had other plans.

Within three months I was hiring a receptionist. In six to nine months, I had two rehab technicians, and by a year or so, I had my first PT assistant. By treating people the way I wanted to treat them, with hands-on or manual style therapy, love, and compassion... my business exploded!

People may not know about physical therapy, or even health care, but they know when they are being treated right, and they spread the word.

Never in a million years did I think I would own my own business. Let alone have 20+ employees, win a Small Business of the Year Award, be the President of the Lillington Chamber of Commerce, conduct interviews for prospective Doctorate of Physical Therapy students at Campbell University, or speak at dozens of community events and groups every year!

God's plan is often different from our own. I thank him for always putting me in the right situation to better follow His plan.

Through the years I have had many trials and tribulations, but He has always provided me with what I need, not what I want, at the exact time I need it. He has put me here to help the people of Harnett County heal, and I have loved every minute of it!

I hope you learn so much from this book. I want everyone to be able to "Improve Your Pelvic Floor, Live Your Life!"

- Sara

CHAPTER 1:
MY PELVIC FLOOR STORY

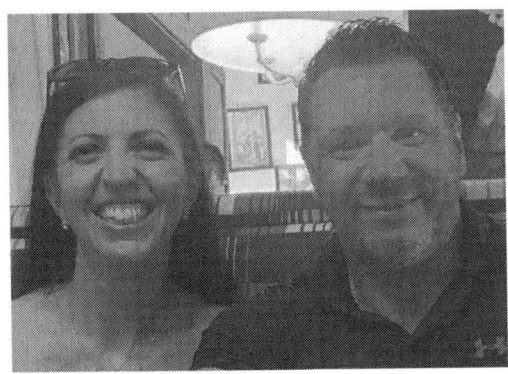

Thirty-three percent of all women under 65 years old suffer from Pelvic Floor Dysfunction. I am one of them. I never knew I had Pelvic Floor Dysfunction. I never knew I had a problem. I believed everything I was experiencing was normal. Then, as I got older, I thought I was just "weird." Finally, I thought something was wrong with me. But, never in my wildest dreams did I think it was a medical condition or that it could be easily fixed!

But let me back up a bit.

When I was young, I leaked urine; not a lot, just a drop here and there. I would notice my underwear was wet, and I would always shove a few pieces of toilet paper in to serve as a pad. In my teenage years, I noticed I leaked more when

I exercised. I thought I was just sweating and that I just sweated a lot in my groin.

I played field hockey in junior high and high school. It wasn't a popular sport, but I loved it! After practices or games, I'd want to go home immediately and change. I remember one time, after a big game, my mom offered to take me out to get hamburgers. I told her I just wanted to go home. What kind of a kid refuses to go out to eat hamburgers??

Subconsciously, I knew I was wet, and I didn't want to "sit in it" for another hour or so.

I could never use tampons. I was deathly afraid of them. They hurt so bad, and I could never get them to work right. And, if I did manage it, I had to take it out within a few minutes because of the pain. But again, I had no idea that this was not normal. So, I never told anyone about it.

When I got married, intercourse was very painful. I'm not talking uncomfortable; I mean painful. I thought I was just different. I didn't know why everyone else enjoyed this, and I had pain with it. It made me feel like a bad wife. It made me feel like there was something wrong with me. It never crossed my mind that it was a medical condition. I wish I had known that a few exercises could save me all that grief!

It turns out I had the classic symptoms of a tight pelvic floor. Many athletic girls/teenagers have tight pelvic floor muscles, and it often goes undiagnosed.

When I was pregnant, things actually got better. The pregnancy stretched out many areas, including my pelvic floor; so much of the pain improved.

During the 3rd trimester, my son sat on the left side of my body for weeks, resulting in horrible back labor pains. Then, he came out on the left side at delivery, rotated my pelvis, and tore the muscles, causing me to get stitches. But, he is a good boy, and he loves his Mama, so it's all good!

After pregnancy and delivery, I leaked if I jumped or coughed. I knew this wasn't normal; I was a Physical Therapist after all, but I thought it would get better as I healed.

A few years after my son was born, my pelvic floor started to tighten back up. I would wake up at least once every night to go to the bathroom, something new for me. Slowly, I started having issues with constipation and fully emptying both my bowel and bladder. At this point, I knew it was an issue. While I wasn't a specialized Pelvic Floor PT at the time, I knew I was experiencing significant problems.

I also knew how Pelvic Floor Physical Therapy worked: internal massage. I was NOT up for that. I told myself I would have to wear a diaper every day before I did that! Also, the closest Pelvic Floor PT was at least an hour away. I couldn't drive that distance and keep working. So, I did what most people do; I ignored it.

In fact, I ignored it until one of my therapists told me she was interested in becoming a Pelvic Floor Physical Therapist. She had suffered from pelvic floor issues in the past, and Pelvic Floor Physical Therapy changed her life. She wanted to help others the way her Pelvic Floor PT helped her. After our conversation, I started doing some research into it. I was absolutely amazed at what I found.

I had no idea how many people suffered from pelvic floor issues. I had no idea how many problems in your body were related to the pelvic floor not working right. I also had no idea that the pelvic floor could be fixed WITHOUT INTERNAL MASSAGE!!! Wow!

Well, you didn't have to tell me twice! I started researching this like crazy. I studied all the pelvic floor training companies until I found one that gave their patients excellent results. They worked on the entire body as a whole functioning unit, not one small area at a time. This concept is also an essential part of our clinic's philosophy (Hence, 'Total Body'). Not only that, but they were able to achieve these amazing results WITHOUT internal work! BINGO!

My therapist and I signed up and never looked back. Then, as I was training, I tried out the techniques on myself. I was amazed at how much of a change I felt.

First, I stopped waking up at night to go to the bathroom. I immediately felt more rested because I was getting solid sleep—my constipation and bloating improved by leaps and bounds, too. (Now I can use the toilet without straining or having difficulty emptying. Yay!) I also noticed that my posture had improved. Soon, I fit into my clothes better, and my stomach and hips began firming up.

I had always been a runner, but apparently, I ran long distances without activating my stomach and hips correctly. I saw a huge difference by using the correct muscles at the right times. I was breathing better, and by improving my breathing pattern, I was getting more air in every breath. My running speed improved just by improving my breathing alone. Even in my same regular workout, I made gains that I had never achieved before. Pelvic Floor Physical Therapy changed my life. And, I have a new passion in life, helping others feel the same way.

I hope you enjoy this book. And if you do, share it with a friend or loved one. After all, they may be one of the millions of people suffering from Pelvic Floor Dysfunction in silence.

- Sara

CHAPTER 2:
WHAT IS THE PELVIC FLOOR?

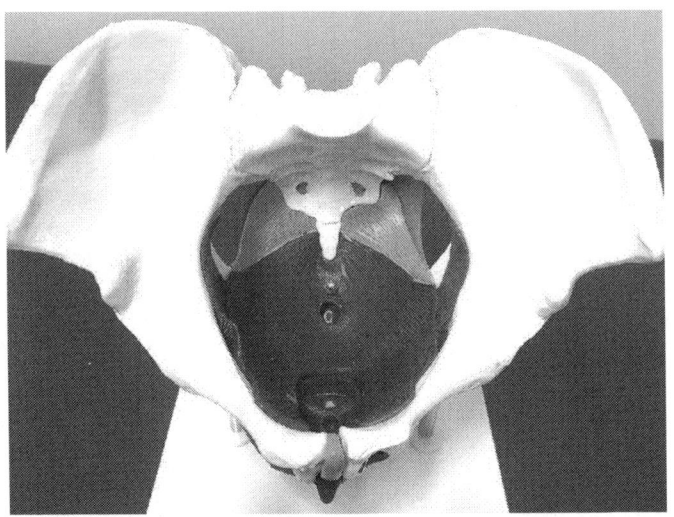

The pelvic floor is made up of several muscles that support the bottom of the pelvis. They stretch from the front of your pelvis, near the top of your groin, to the back of your pelvis, attaching at your tailbone. They also go from side to side and connect in your hip joints. When you hear the term "hip," many people have a different idea of where the hip is. When I use the term "hip joint," I am referring to the ball and socket joint on the outside of your thigh. You can think of the pelvic floor as a sling or a hammock of muscles that sits below the pelvis. Both men and women have pelvic floors.

What Does the Pelvic Floor Do?

The pelvic floor muscles have two main jobs:

- To support your organs
- To control your bowel and bladder

Supporting Your Organs:

You have many organs in your abdominal area. They are supported in the front by your abdominal or belly muscles and in the back by your lower back muscles. In addition, the pelvic floor supports them from the bottom and must hold the weight of the organs themselves. As your body builds up urine in your bladder, the weight of that urine gets heavier. The pelvic floor muscles must work harder to hold the heavier weight. After you go to the bathroom and urinate, they have less weight to support and need to work less. However, as with any muscle, they can only hold so much weight. When the urine weight is too much for the pelvic floor muscles to hold, leaking can occur. We will get more into this in later chapters.

Controlling Your Bowel and Bladder:

The pelvic floor muscles hold in your bowels (stool or poop) and bladder (urine or pee). When you go to the bathroom and are ready to release your bowels or bladder, your pelvic floor muscles need to relax to allow for the emptying to occur. When you finish using the bathroom, they need to contract and return to holding in the bowel and bladder.

As well as being strong and flexible, your pelvic floor muscles need to be coordinated. Nine muscles make up the pelvic floor. They must work in the correct sequence to function properly. The pelvic floor must relax to allow for urination, bowel movements, and sexual intercourse.

Coordinated contracting and relaxing of the pelvic floor muscles is needed to control bowel and bladder functions.

Pelvic Floor Dysfunction happens when there is too much tension on the pelvic floor muscles (high tone) or not enough (low tone). Issues also occur when the muscles do not know when to contract or relax properly or are unable to contract and relax properly. These problems can contribute to a host of symptoms, including urinary incontinence, constipation, pain during intercourse, inability to achieve an erection, or pain in the lower back, pelvic region, genitals, or rectum.

CHAPTER 3:
WHAT CAUSES THE PELVIC FLOOR NOT TO WORK CORRECTLY?

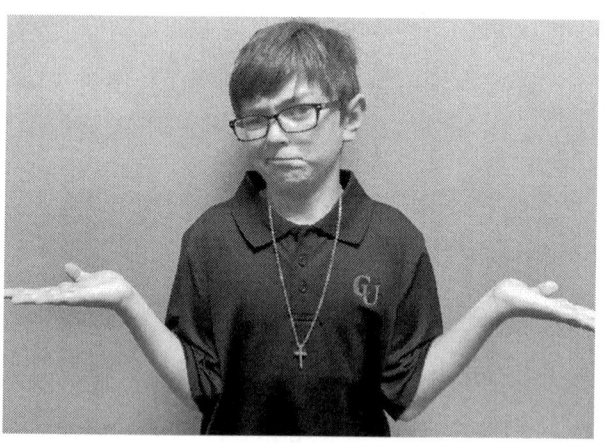

Many issues can cause your pelvic floor to work improperly. This problem is called Pelvic Floor Dysfunction (PFD).

Reasons for PFD Include:

- Traumatic injuries to the pelvic area (like a car accident or sexual assault)
- Pregnancy
- Overusing the pelvic muscles
- Pelvic surgery (including abdominal or reproductive organs)
- Being overweight

- Advancing age
- Menopause
- Gastric reflux
- Hernia

Does Pregnancy Cause Pelvic Floor Dysfunction?

Pregnancy is a common cause of Pelvic Floor Dysfunction. Twenty-five percent of women with vaginal deliveries without any complications experience Pelvic Floor Dysfunction. If there are any complications, the chances of Pelvic Floor Dysfunction increase.

Pelvic Floor Dysfunction Chances Increase with:

- Tearing or episiotomy
- A prolonged pushing phase of labor
- Vacuum, forceps, or other emergency procedures
- Delivering multiple babies at once (twins, triplets, etc.)
- Excessive weight gain during pregnancy
- Having multiple pregnancies (the more children you have, the higher your chances of having Pelvic Floor Dysfunction)

It is important to realize that you can have Pelvic Floor Dysfunction even with a C-section. The C-section cuts into your belly muscles, and the baby does not exit through the pelvic floor. This lessens the chance of damage to your pelvic floor during the birthing process. But remember, your pelvic floor muscles and tissues become strained during pregnancy itself! So, it's not just the baby leaving your body; carrying the baby stretches and strains the pelvic floor muscles as well.

Now, let me ask you another question: WHY did you NEED the C-section in the first place? Many women require a Cesarean because the baby cannot be delivered vaginally. If you push and push and the baby can't come out, you have still strained (and possibly injured) your pelvic floor. So yes, Pelvic Floor Dysfunction can still happen with a Cesarean section.

Other Reasons for Pelvic Floor Dysfunction:
We can't blame it all on the kids! There are many different reasons why Pelvic Floor Dysfunction occurs. Any abdominal surgery can affect your pelvic floor. We will get into this more in later chapters when we talk about pressure in your abdomen or trunk.

Think About This:

The pelvic floor supports your pelvis from the BOTTOM. What supports it in the FRONT? That's right, your abdomen or belly muscles. If you have weakness, scar tissue, surgical scars, or other issues with your belly muscles, they cannot do their job as well. If the abdominal muscles are not holding the pelvis up at the front, the posture of the pelvis changes. The pelvis can tilt forward in the front, causing the pelvic floor muscles underneath to tighten or cramp up.

With the belly muscles not supporting your organs in the front, your pelvic floor muscles have to work harder to support the pelvis to compensate for the weakness in that area. This constant overworking can also cause pelvic floor problems.

Constipation:

When constipated, you may have to push harder to get your stool (bowels or poop) out. Constipation can also cause you to change positions on the toilet or use your hand to help eliminate stool. It's thought that up to half of people suffering from long-term constipation also have Pelvic Floor Dysfunction.

There are many reasons for constipation, but the result is always the same. The frequent and prolonged pushing pressure can damage and strain your pelvic floor. In addition, frequent constipation can have a lasting effect on the pelvic floor muscles and cause them to be too weak from constant pushing against them. This leads to Pelvic Floor Dysfunction.

Constant straining and pushing can also lead to Pelvic Organ Prolapse (POP). POP is when your internal organs start sliding down. At first, Pelvic Organ Prolapse is not noticeable. However, as it progresses through the stages, it may become so bad that you can see and feel your organs on the outside of your body. Prolapse can happen to your bladder, vagina, or rectum. We will talk more about Pelvic Organ Prolapse later in the book. In general, I consider Pelvic Organ Prolapse to be "bad." We should try anything we can to avoid it!

Diarrhea:

On the other end of the spectrum, going to the bathroom too often can also cause Pelvic Floor Dysfunction. This is because each time you go to the bathroom, you are asking your pelvic floor muscles to loosen. Frequent overuse of these muscles may eventually lead to poor muscle coordination. This occurs when the pelvic floor muscles become confused and do not know when to contract and relax properly. This dysfunction often leads to the inability to control your bowels and the immediate need to RUN to the bathroom to avoid an accident. Over time this can worsen, leading to fecal incontinence.

Is Pelvic Floor Dysfunction Hereditary?
Pelvic Floor Dysfunction is a hereditary condition, meaning it can run in families. Researchers are looking into a potential genetic cause of this dysfunction.

CHAPTER 4:
WHAT DOES PELVIC FLOOR DYSFUNCTION FEEL LIKE?

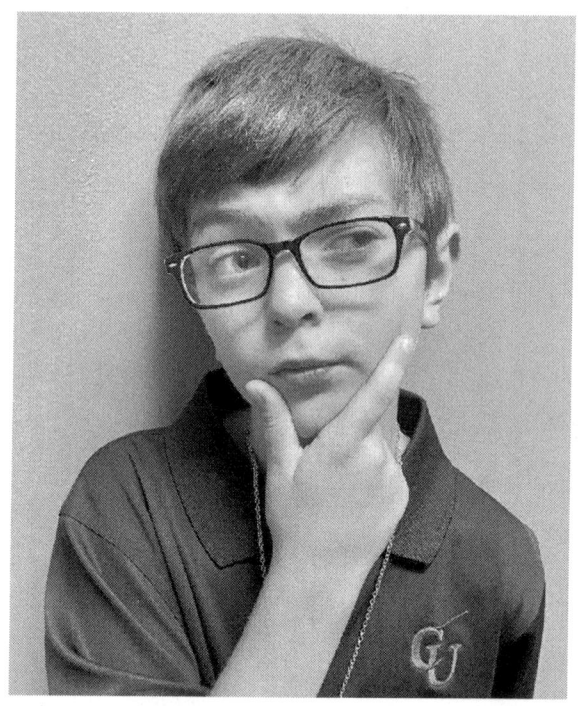

Several Symptoms May Be a Sign That You Have Pelvic Floor Dysfunction.

If you have any of these symptoms, you should discuss them with a Pelvic Floor Specialist:

- Frequently needing to use the bathroom; you may also feel like you need to 'force it out' to go, or you might stop and start many times

- Constipation: It's thought that up to half of people suffering from long-term constipation also have Pelvic Floor Dysfunction
- Straining or pushing hard to pass a bowel movement, or having to change positions on the toilet or use your hand to help eliminate stool
- Have difficulty starting to urinate or emptying the bladder completely
- Leaking stool or urine; this may be as little as one drop or as much as a full bladder
- Leak urine when coughing, laughing, or exercising
- Leak stool or have difficulty controlling gas
- Have difficulty making it to the bathroom in time
- Painful urination
- Pain during sex
- Feeling pain in your lower back with no other cause
- Feeling ongoing pain in your pelvic region, genitals, or rectum — with or without having a bowel movement

- Feel heaviness, fullness, pulling, or aching in the vagina that worsens by the end of the day or is related to a bowel movement
- You see or feel a 'bulge' or 'something coming out' of the vagina

Is Pelvic Floor Dysfunction Different for Men and Women?

There are different pelvic conditions that are unique to men and women. In the next few chapters, we will address these.

CHAPTER 5:
PELVIC FLOOR DYSFUNCTION IN MEN

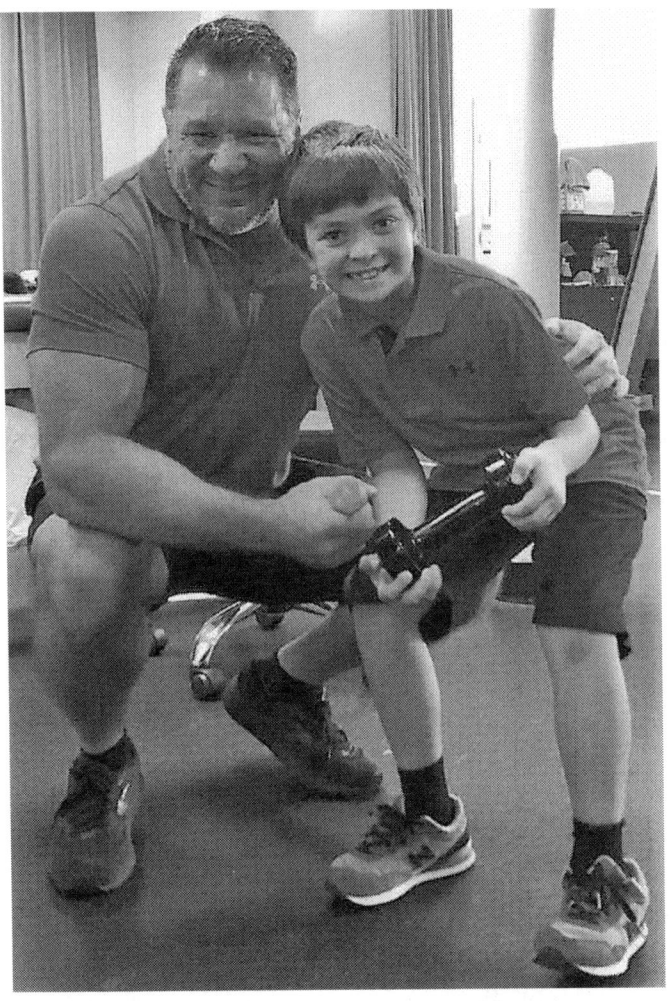

I know what you are thinking, and the answer is 'yes.' Yes, men have pelvic floors, too. However, most people have no idea that men, as well as women, have pelvic floors. For a long time, I was one of them! And if men do not know that they have a pelvic floor, how are they supposed to know if there is something wrong with their pelvic floor?

So, if men have pelvic floors, what does the pelvic floor do?

The Role of the Pelvic Floor Muscles in Men:
1. Support and stabilize the organs
2. Controls the releasing and holding of the bowel and bladder
3. Sexual function
4. Help with breathing and respiration
5. Stabilize and provide balance

Every year, millions of men around the world experience Pelvic Floor Dysfunction. This is because the pelvic floor muscles work as part of the waste and reproductive systems. Because they work in both areas, Pelvic Floor Dysfunction can co-exist with many other conditions affecting men.

These Include:
- Male urinary dysfunction
- Male bowel dysfunction

- Prostatitis
- Erectile dysfunction

Male Urinary Dysfunction - This Condition Can Involve:

- Leaking urine after you have stopped peeing.

- Leaking after more vigorous activities such as jumping, running, or coughing is known as Stress Incontinence.

- Leaking with prolonged activity. Many men tell me they do not leak unless they walk or are active for over 30 minutes. This means the muscles are strong enough to support them for 30 minutes. After that, they can no longer support the bladder. Once they are fatigued, leaking occurs.

- Urge to run to the bathroom "right now" as soon as the sensation occurs. Once you feel the need to urinate, the muscles have a very short time that they can work properly and hold in the bladder. Then leaking occurs. This is known as Urge Incontinence.

- Tightness in pelvic floor muscles can cause pain, spasms, or the inability to empty your bowel or bladder when using the toilet. Many men feel the urge to urinate, but when they get to the bathroom, little to nothing comes out.

Male Bowel Dysfunction:

Muscles in the rectum and anus control releasing and holding in your stool. When the muscles of the anus contract, they tighten up and prevent feces from being released. The relaxing of these muscles allows the anus to open and the feces to be removed. When the muscles have difficulty holding or staying contracted when needed, the result can be bowel incontinence. This can range from leaking a small amount of feces when you do a particular activity to as much as fully emptying the bowels at unwanted times.

If your body cannot fully hold a contraction of your anus muscles when needed, the result can be releasing bowels at unwanted times. If you cannot fully contract or close the anus muscles after you are finished on the toilet, leaking can happen shortly afterward. Both can end with embarrassment and messy clothes. On the other end of the spectrum, constipation can occur if you cannot relax the anus muscles when trying to empty your bowels. Often people will experience the sensation that they cannot fully empty their bowels. In other words, "you still have to go after you go." This can be due to the tightness of the pelvic floor muscles. When the pelvic floor muscles are too tight, they often have trouble relaxing. This can cause constipation and/or the inability to fully empty your bowels.

In addition to needing the correct amount of strength and relaxation in these muscles, coordination is also important. Your muscles need to know when and how to contract and relax when you tell them to do so.

Bowel Incontinence May Be Caused by Things Such as:

- Diarrhea
- Constipation
- Damage to the nervous system from disease or injury
- Rectum bulging down into the anus (rectal prolapse)
- Crohn's disease or ulcerative colitis

Stool Leakage/Incontinence Can Be Caused by Factors Other Than Your Pelvic Floor, Such as:

- Medicine side effects
- Stress
- Multiple sclerosis
- Stroke

- Alzheimer's disease
- Diabetes
- Infections, including spinal cord or brain infections
- Hemorrhoids
- Damage after surgery

As with many issues, bowel incontinence or leaking has many causes. Make sure to mention this to your primary care provider.

Prostatitis:

Pelvic Floor Dysfunction symptoms closely resemble prostatitis, an infection or inflammation of the prostate (a male reproductive gland). Prostatitis can have many causes, including bacteria, sexually transmitted infections, or trauma to the nervous system. Therefore, it is important to speak with your Primary Care Physician (PCP) or Urologist if you exhibit inflammation in the penis or prostate as you may need other treatment.

Erectile Dysfunction (ED) or Impotence:

Erectile dysfunction is when men cannot achieve or maintain an erection firm enough for intercourse. Thirty million men in the United States suffer from ED. In fact, one out of ten men will suffer from ED at some point in their lifetime. Therefore, occasional ED is not uncommon. However, if ED occurs more than 50% of the time, it can indicate a medical issue.

Unfortunately, ED is often associated with reduced sexual activity, low self-esteem, strain on the relationship with one's partner, and depression. Depression and erectile dysfunction are very intertwined. It is shown that depression can lead to ED, and ED can also lead to depression. Men that suffer from ED are three times more likely to experience depression than those without it. Men that suffer from ED are also two times more likely to suffer from a stroke or a heart attack. Seventy-nine percent (79%) of men that suffer from ED are also obese.

Many factors contribute to ED.

Factors That Contribute to Erectile Dysfunction (ED) or Impotence:

- Advancing age
- Anxiety/depression
- Constipation
- Diabetes

- Generalized poor health
- Heart disease
- High cholesterol
- Illicit drug use
- Long-term, persistent coughing (such as smoker's cough, bronchitis, or asthma)
- Low testosterone levels
- Medication
- Multiple sclerosis
- Overweight
- Parkinson's disease
- Pelvic floor weakness
- Persistent heavy lifting
- Prolonged inactivity
- Prostate cancer or prostate surgery
- Reduced blood flow
- Sleep disorders
- Smoking

- Stress
- Surgery for bladder or bowel problems

Wow, that's a long list! Pelvic muscle tension, weakness, or pain can often contribute to the cause of ED. The muscles that lift the penis and maintain an erection are part of the pelvic floor. So, if your pelvic floor muscles are weak, they may not be able to lift and/or hold the penis to achieve or maintain an erection. If the pelvic floor muscles are tight, they cannot activate properly to achieve an erection. If one of these is the case, exercise is highly effective in improving erectile dysfunction.

Reasons the Male Pelvic Floor Muscles May Become Weak:

- Acid reflux
- Chronic coughing (COPD, emphysema, asthma, etc.)
- Constipation
- Diarrhea
- Inactivity
- Prostate cancer or prostate surgery
- Surgery in the abdomen or pelvis
- Scar tissue

We will learn about this in later chapters, but many of these issues alter the abdomen and pelvic floor pressure. When more pressure is placed on the pelvic floor muscles, it can cause leakage, weakness, spasms, pain, and/or ED. Make sure to read the chapter on pressure for more information.

How Do We Know That Exercise is Helpful for Erectile Dysfunction?

One research study by Professor Grace Dorey aimed to test the effectiveness of pelvic floor muscle exercise on men with erectile dysfunction. They took fifty-five men with erectile dysfunction whose ED was not due to surgery but from other causes. The control group did not exercise, while the Intervention group performed pelvic floor muscle exercises: three sets a day, every day, for three months.

No improvement was found in the group without exercise. However, the study found that doing three sets of pelvic floor muscle exercises every day for three months improved ED in 75% of men!

- 40% of men felt that they were 'cured'
- 35% of men felt that they 'improved to satisfaction'

In fact, after the study, the intervention group (that performed pelvic floor exercises) did so well that the researchers gave the control group the same exercises to do for three more months. The trend continued, and the control group improved ED by 76% as well!

Exercise has a significant effect on erectile dysfunction. It is also beneficial for many of the conditions that can cause ED (depression, anxiety, diabetes, cardiac issues, obesity, and many more!) So, it makes sense if exercise is helpful for ED alone, and that exercise is helpful for the conditions that can cause the ED, exercise is a good choice of treatment. Like anything else you often need to combine exercise with other treatment(s) you may be receiving for ED.

Let's Look at One Example:
There is a man with high blood pressure and poor circulation. He also has erectile dysfunction. So yes, these medical issues can contribute to or cause ED. But that does not mean that he doesn't ALSO have pelvic floor muscle weakness. A pelvic floor physical therapy examination will be ideal to see if the pelvic floor muscles are contributing to ED. Often it is not one magic pill that makes a difference in controlling erectile dysfunction. Instead, it is a combination of treatments.

You may have high blood pressure and poor circulation. Yes, these can contribute to or cause ED. But that does not mean that you don't ALSO have pelvic floor muscle weakness.

Let Me Ask You a Few Questions:

Q: What is the usual treatment for most erectile dysfunction?

A: *You got it - Medicine.*

Q: What is the usual treatment for Pelvic Floor Dysfunction?

A: *Exercise.*

Q: Which one of those treatments have a higher chance of harming you? Which one of those treatments have a higher chance of an adverse side effect?

A: *As we all know, medication has much higher chances of adverse side effects than exercise, especially if exercise is supervised by a professional.*

Now Answer This:

Q: Which one of those things will be good for you regardless of whether it is the answer to your erectile dysfunction or not?

A: *(Hint: It's EXERCISE!)*

Pelvic floor muscle weakness is often a contributing factor to erectile dysfunction. That means even if you know that you have some medical issues causing erectile dysfunction, you can still have pelvic floor muscle weakness. However, adding pelvic floor muscle exercises can result in a longer, stronger erection with or without medication. And that's the goal.

That's why many providers and specialists are prescribing pelvic floor muscle exercises FIRST, even before medicine, to see if that will solve the problem.

If exercise doesn't work or solve it completely, only then will they add medication.

It is important to remember that building muscle takes time. You do not walk into the gym with a potbelly and expect to step out of the gym looking like Arnold Schwarzenegger in one day. Of course not! Muscles take time to strengthen and develop. So, it should not come as a surprise that your pelvic floor muscles are no different.

However, pelvic floor muscle exercises MUST BE DONE CONSISTENTLY for three to six weeks to see results.

Did you read that???

Because it is so important, I'm going to write it again.

Pelvic floor muscle exercises MUST BE DONE CONSISTENTLY for three to six weeks to see results. If a person stops doing the exercises, the muscles may weaken, and leakage and/or erectile dysfunction may return.

So be consistent. <u>Be patient</u>! Hang in there! Don't give up on one of the most successful, natural, and beneficial treatments out there!

Other Types of Exercise That Can Help:
Since erectile dysfunction can also be due to other aspects of health, working on your overall health has been proven to help symptoms. For example, aerobic exercise can also benefit people with ED. Research studies showed that men who practiced an aerobic (cardiovascular) exercise four times a week saw the best results (according to the authors of a 2018 systematic research review).

Each exercise session, you should work up to a goal of moderate or high-intensity that lasts a minimum of forty minutes. In addition, a person should keep up their aerobic exercise routine for at least six months.

Some Examples of Aerobic Exercises Include:
- Cycling
- Spin classes
- Boxing
- Running
- Rowing
- Walking

Improving the Diet:
Diet and weight loss are also important aspects of ED treatment and prevention. Following dietary guidelines and limiting the intake of alcohol, tobacco, and foods with added salt, sugar, and fat have been proven to help reduce the risk of developing ED. These efforts can also reduce the risk of strokes, metabolic diseases, and cardiovascular diseases linked to ED.

Erectile dysfunction (ED) is a complex condition, so Pelvic Floor Dysfunction may or may not be the sole cause. Other issues like smoking, high blood pressure, or decreased circulation may contribute to ED. Be sure to talk with your physician and see if adding pelvic floor exercise will be helpful for you.

PROSTATE CANCER & PROSTATE SURGERY:

Throughout the world, one out of six men will develop prostate cancer. That's a pretty high statistic, so it is vital that men know the risks and side effects. If you are diagnosed with prostate cancer, your doctor will talk about your treatment options. Unfortunately, due to the location of the prostate, many treatments can have side effects that affect the function of the pelvic floor. Unfortunately, many of these side effects can significantly affect the quality of life for men.

Side Effects of Prostate Cancer Treatment May Include:
1. Bladder leakage
2. Bowel leakage
3. Erectile dysfunction

With a prostatectomy, much or all the prostate is removed. Due to its location, injury to the surrounding muscles and/or nerves may occur. Additionally, the pelvic floor muscles in men are not as thick as they are in women. For this reason, incontinence in men can be more severe. Many men will leak larger amounts of urine and/or stool than women. This can be very embarrassing, often resulting in limiting activities or the number of times a person leaves their home.

As the day progresses and muscles fatigue, leakage symptoms are likely to worsen. Exercise for the pelvic floor muscles can improve the blood flow to this area and expedite healing. It can also strengthen these muscles to contract and relax more efficiently. Strengthening the pelvic floor muscles can improve bowel and bladder leakage and improvement in ED.

What Does Urinary Incontinence Look Like for Men Who Have Undergone Radical Prostatectomy?
Leaking with:

- Standing up or with large movements
- 'Breaking wind'
- Coughing, sneezing, or laughing
- Lifting, bending, or squatting
- Before or after urination
- In the afternoon, when your muscles get tired
- You hear water: water taps, shower, hoses, etc.
- Caffeine consumption

- Alcohol consumption, especially beer
- Sexual arousal

What Does Bowel Dysfunction Look Like for Men Who Have Undergone Radical Prostatectomy?

- Diarrhea
- Constipation
- Leakage of bowels
- Inability to control bowels
- Leaking bowels when 'breaking wind'
- Urgency: "I gotta go right now!"
- Rectal bleeding

The issues above can range from mild to severe and are different from person to person. While the problems mentioned can be due to various things, pelvic floor muscle weakness or tightness can be a culprit. Even if another medical issue is found to be the cause of your symptoms, Pelvic Floor Muscle Dysfunction often co-exists and makes the symptoms worse. If you experience any of these symptoms, be sure to contact your provider. Also, be sure to ask if Pelvic Floor Physical Therapy, in conjunction with other treatments, may be right for you.

CHAPTER 6:
PELVIC FLOOR DYSFUNCTION IN WOMEN

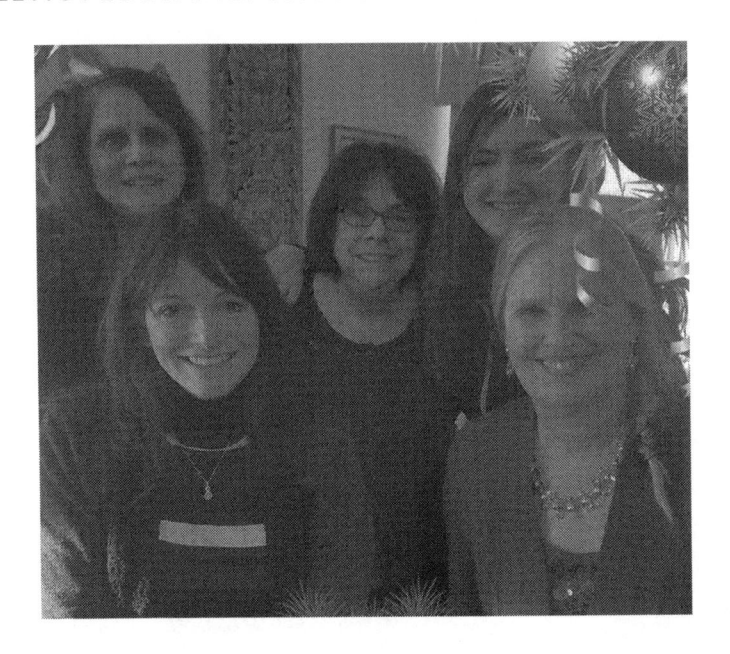

Pelvic Floor Dysfunction can have different symptoms in women than in men. These symptoms may interfere with a woman's reproductive health by affecting the uterus and vagina. Women who get Pelvic Floor Dysfunction may also have other symptoms like pain during intercourse or difficulty using a tampon. One out of four women (25%) twenty years or older suffer from Pelvic Floor Dysfunction. They often struggle with one or more symptoms, including Pelvic Organ Prolapse (POP), Urinary Incontinence (UI), and

Fecal Incontinence (FI, also called Anal Incontinence or Accidental Bowel Leakage).

Let's look at how Pelvic Floor Dysfunctions can affect women of various age groups.

Teenage Years:

As if teenage years aren't hard enough, it's also a time when girls can suffer in silence from Pelvic Floor Dysfunction. Some people have pelvic floor muscles that are too tight and cannot relax. This can be made worse by doing squeezing exercises and overworking the muscles without learning how to relax.

Often this occurs with very active or athletic girls. Active young girls are constantly using their muscles. The muscles can often work without issue but do not know how to relax properly. This constant tightening of pelvic floor muscles without relaxing may cause prolonged pain and tightness.

Think of it as a cramp. For example, if your muscles keep working and working and never relax, they may cramp up. Similarly, the pelvic floor muscles can work and work without relaxing. Then they finally "cramp up." This is especially common in teenage girls if they play more than one sport throughout the year or are very active for more than just a few months a year.

This cramping of the pelvic floor may result in obstruction of the bowels or bladder, incontinence, constipation, pain/irritation with urination, or pain when moving your bowels. Some teens may also be under treatment for recurrent urinary tract infections (UTIs).

Pregnancy/Childbirth:

During pregnancy, your uterus is slowly growing day by day to hold your wonderful baby! As that beautiful baby continues to grow, he gets heavier and heavier. After nine months of excess pressure weighing down on your pelvic floor muscles, there is no wonder that this can injure the muscles holding in the baby! No matter your birthing story, it is important to remember that injury can occur during pregnancy.

Childbirth itself can also injure the pelvic floor. When I say childbirth, I mean labor, the pushing part. If you've ever had a baby vaginally, I don't suppose I have to explain how this can stretch things out and cause injury! (And if you haven't had a baby vaginally, I am sure you can imagine).

Childbirth can contribute to the development of Pelvic Floor Disorders because it may put excessive strain on the pelvic floor during delivery. For example, vaginal births double the rate of Pelvic Floor Disorders compared to Cesarean deliveries or women who never gave birth. And the more births you have, the more your chances of Pelvic Floor Disorders increase.

Menopause:

During menopause, women produce lower amounts of estrogen. This hormone does many different things for our body, so you can expect various symptoms when you have low levels. For example, one of the things estrogen does is help to make our muscles strong. However, when we are low on estrogen, all our muscles become weak. If you are stronger going into menopause or pre-menopause, you will have less difficulty with this.

But if you already have weak areas, you may develop problems in those areas when you enter menopause. In addition, if you have had multiple children or are at a higher risk for pelvic floor injury and never had pelvic floor symptoms, weakening your muscles even further may be enough to start experiencing symptoms.

The Pelvic Floor Muscles Often Weaken During Menopause, Which Can Lead to Many Symptoms We Have Already Discussed:

- Frequently needing to use the bathroom

- Constipation
- Straining or pushing hard to pass a bowel movement
- Leaking stool or urine
- Painful urination
- Pain during intercourse
- Feeling pain in your lower back with no other cause
- Feeling ongoing pain or heaviness in your pelvic region, genitals, or rectum — with or without a bowel movement

Pelvic floor muscle weakness can also lead to Pelvic Organ Prolapse (POP). Pelvic floor muscle weakness is very different from Pelvic Organ Prolapse. Pelvic Organ Prolapse happens when the muscles holding a woman's pelvic organs (uterus, rectum, and bladder) in place loosens and becomes too stretched out. Pelvic Organ Prolapse can cause the organs to protrude (stick out) of the vagina or rectum. Initially, POP may cause a "heavy" feeling in the groin area. As prolapse progresses, you may be able to feel your organs with your fingers or even see them.

The Symptoms of Pelvic Organ Prolapse Are:
- Feeling heaviness, fullness, pulling, or aching in the vagina that gets worse by the end of the day or is related to a bowel movement
- Seeing or feeling a 'bulge' or 'something coming out' of the vagina
- Having difficulty starting to urinate or emptying the bladder completely
- Leaking urine when coughing, laughing, or exercising
- Leaking stool or have difficulty controlling gas
- Having difficulty making it to the bathroom in time

Senior Citizen:

Once you have passed through menopause (and are finally done with hot flashes, night sweats, and all the other fun stuff), many seniors can continue to have their muscles weaken. In addition, the strength of the pelvic floor deteriorates as women age, which can also lead to the development of POP.

CHAPTER 7:
OTHER FACTORS THAT INCREASE PELVIC FLOOR DYSFUNCTION

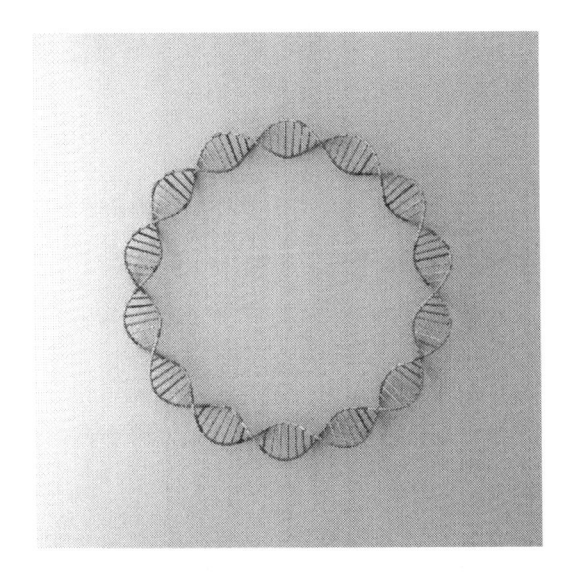

Although pregnancy and delivery commonly cause pelvic floor issues, we can't blame it all on the babies! Many other factors can increase your risk of Pelvic Floor Dysfunction.

Genetic:

Some people are born with weaker pelvic floor muscles, which puts them at a greater risk for Pelvic Floor Dysfunction. Also, if your mother or sister has a PFD, you are at a higher risk of developing one.

Race:

Caucasian women are more likely to develop prolapse and to have urine leakage related to coughing, sneezing, and activities. African American women are more likely to have urinary leakage related to urgency.

Ethnicity:

Mexican American women are more likely to struggle with urinary incontinence than other Hispanic/Latino women. However, this difference may reflect a reluctance to seek medical care or a language barrier.

Lifestyles That Can Affect Your Chances of Pelvic Floor Dysfunctions:

Obesity:

Being overweight or obese places increased pressure on the bladder. It often goes hand in hand with a lack of strength in pelvic and core muscles. As a result, overweight people have an increased risk of developing POP and Urinary Incontinence (UI).

Diet:

When there is not enough fiber or water in a person's diet, bowel movements are more likely to be hard or irregular. In addition, processed foods can lead to constipation. Certain foods also can irritate the bladder, making people feel like they have the urge to urinate. Bladder irritants include caffeine and alcohol.

Smoking:

Women who smoke increase their risk of developing POP and UI. In addition, smoking is generally not good for bladder health. It also can damage the connective tissue in your body, including the tissue in your pelvic area.

Heavy Lifting/Exertion:

Certain occupations, usually those that involve heavy lifting or exertion, can increase the risk of developing PFDs. In addition, repetitive strenuous activity is also a risk. For example, for some people, stair climbing can cause leakage.

Health Problems/Medical History That Can Cause Pelvic Floor Dysfunctions:

Constipation/Chronic Straining:

Straining with constipation places significant pressure on the weak vaginal wall and can further thin it out. This increases the risk for Pelvic Floor Dysfunction or prolapse. Any medical condition that causes more constipation can also increase your risk of developing a pelvic floor injury. This is true for males or females.

Pelvic Injury/Surgery:

Loss of pelvic support can occur when the pelvic floor is injured from falls, car accidents, or surgery. Injuries can cause scar tissue to build up in the abdomen and pelvis, whether you have had surgery in the area or not. Scar tissue can bind down muscles and prevent them from working correctly. They can pull on structures or organs from the inside and cause pain or other symptoms. In addition, abdominal surgeries, hysterectomy, and other abdominal procedures that treat Pelvic Organ Prolapse can sometimes cause further prolapse.

Lung Conditions/Chronic Coughing:

Chronic respiratory disorders can cause increased pressure in the abdomen and pelvis during coughing. If you have any condition which causes you to cough more frequently, this can also increase your risk of Pelvic Floor Dysfunction and/or Pelvic Organ Prolapse. These can include but are not limited to:

- Allergies
- Asthma
- Chronic Obstructive Pulmonary Disorder (COPD)
- Gastroesophageal Reflux Disease (GERD)

- Medications
- Smoking

Sexual Dysfunction:

Pelvic floor symptoms are significantly associated with reduced sexual arousal, infrequent orgasm, and painful intercourse (known in medical terms as dyspareunia). Often this can be due to pelvic floor muscle tightness. Some people immediately experience pain during sexual intercourse, while some have pain after a certain amount of time.

Some women tell me they feel as if their "vagina has closed up." When you feel this way, there is a high chance that your pelvic floor muscles are tight. When your muscles become tight, they become smaller. As a result, the opening to your vagina may be smaller, perhaps giving the sensation that it is "closed up." Pelvic Floor Physical Therapy is very successful at improving muscle tightness in the pelvic region! Keep reading for more details.

**If you do have pain during intercourse, be sure to discuss it with your physician as well.

Health Conditions or Injuries That Affect the Nerves:
For example, diabetes, Parkinson's Disease, stroke, back surgery, spinal stenosis, or childbirth can weaken the pelvic floor muscles.

Emotional Stress:
Emotional stress can make you feel anxious and that you need to go to the bathroom more often. For some, it can also result in loose stools, for others, constipation. Several areas in the body tend to 'store stress.' For example, does your neck ever get tight when you are stressed? Or maybe your lower back? Well, your pelvic floor is another one of those areas that tend to tighten up as we stress. It is very common for tightness and pelvic floor symptoms to worsen during emotional stress.

If you have one or more of the factors listed above, it is important to control them the best you can. By doing this, you can lower your risk of Pelvic Floor Dysfunction. Some of these things you will have more control over than others. For example, you have little control over your genetics. But you do have control over your diet. You can change that. Perhaps you have one of the medical conditions above. Let's take asthma. You cannot get rid of asthma (Don't we wish!), but you can get it under control to the best of your ability by following up with your provider regularly. You may still be at a higher risk of Pelvic Floor Dysfunction, but you can lower the risk as much as possible.

CHAPTER 8:
INCONTINENCE MYTHS

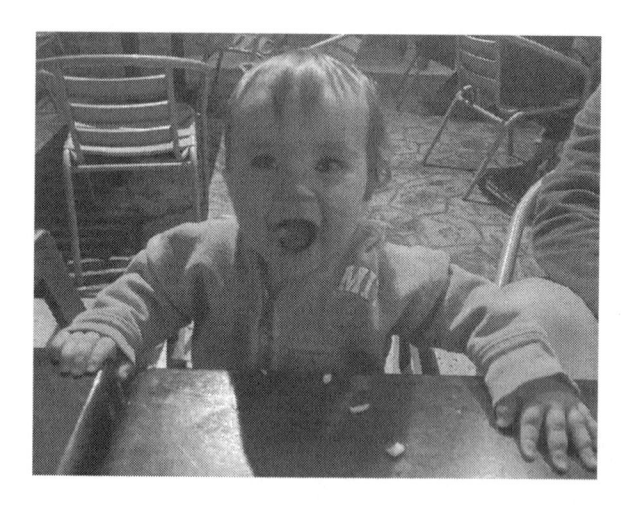

Do you have incontinence? Do you know someone who does? I think you'll be surprised to find out just how common incontinence is. What throws off many people is that they do not know what incontinence truly means in medical terms.

Let Me Start with Defining Incontinence:
Incontinence is the loss of bladder or bowel control. Period. It doesn't mean you wake up at night with your bed soaking wet (although it could). It doesn't necessarily mean that you have no control over your bladder. It doesn't mean that you wear an adult diaper all day, every day. It simply means that, at times, you lose urine or bowels without having control

over it. It can range anywhere from a drop when you sneeze or cough, needing to go "Right NOW!" when you feel the sensation, or even to emptying your entire bladder when you stand up.

So, let me ask you again, do you suffer from incontinence?

There are two myths about incontinence that drive me crazy. So, before we even start, we are going to debunk them now.

Common Incontinence Myths:

1. Leaking is normal after having a baby
2. Leaking is normal as you get older

No. No, No, and No!

Leaking or incontinence is COMMON after having a baby.

Leaking or incontinence is COMMON as we age.

But that does not mean it is *normal* or that you have to put up with it.

Urinary incontinence (the loss of bladder control) is a common and often embarrassing problem.

In July of 2018, the Mayo Clinic found that urinary incontinence affects one in four women under 65. One out of four! That's 25% of all women! Furthermore, the prevalence of this problem increases with age. Up to 75% of women above the age of 65 report urine leakage. (WOW!)

The severity ranges from occasionally leaking urine when you cough or sneeze to having an urge to urinate that's so sudden and strong you don't get to a toilet in time.

Urinary incontinence frequently occurs during pregnancy or after childbirth. But remember, just because it is common does not mean it is normal. Though it happens more often as people get older, urinary incontinence IS NOT a normal part of aging. If urinary incontinence affects your daily activities, don't hesitate to see your doctor or a Pelvic Floor Physical Therapist. For most people, simple exercises, lifestyle and dietary changes, or medical care can treat symptoms of urinary incontinence.

If incontinence is an issue for you, it is important to remember that it is treatable. No matter how extreme or minimal the leaking is, it signifies that there is a problem elsewhere in your body. Treatment is safe, effective, and simple. Best yet, it can be done with specialized exercises and stretching. No one even needs to touch your pelvic floor!

Question to Think About:

"How would your life change if you did not have to worry about leaking or making it to the toilet in time?"

CHAPTER 9:
TYPES OF INCONTINENCE

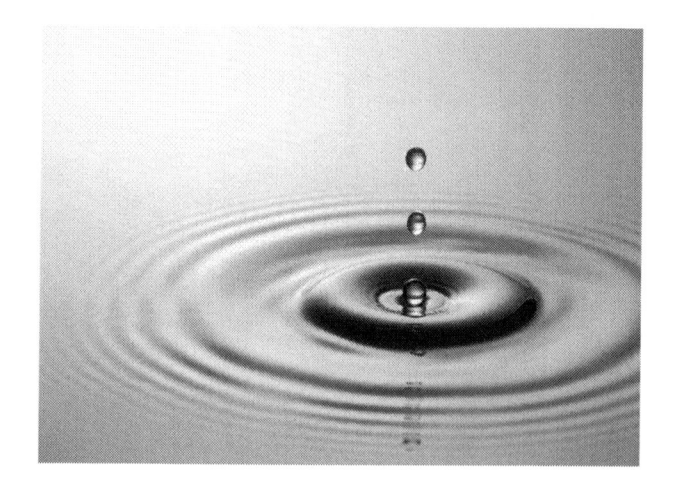

Many people experience occasional, minor leaks of urine. Others may lose small to moderate amounts of urine more frequently. Others still experience complete emptying of their bowels or bladders when doing certain activities. There are many types of incontinence. Each type shows when leaking is most likely to happen.

It's important to determine the type of urinary incontinence that you have. Just like anything else, the treatment changes based on your exact type of incontinence. Your symptoms often tell your Pelvic Health Provider which type you have. That information, as well as your physical presentation, will help your Pelvic Floor Specialist determine the best care for you.

Types of Urinary Incontinence Include:
- Stress Incontinence
- Urge Incontinence
- Overflow Incontinence
- Functional Incontinence
- Mixed Incontinence

It is important to diagnose which kind of incontinence you are suffering from. Like most things, each of these are treated differently. And yes, there ARE treatments for all of these.

SPOILER ALERT: Successful treatment doesn't involve medicine or surgery!

Stress Incontinence:
Urine leaks when you exert pressure on your bladder. This is most common with coughing, sneezing, laughing, exercising, or lifting something heavy. When you perform these activities, your body increases the pressure in your trunk to accomplish them. This places more pressure directly onto your pelvic floor. If you leak when you cough, sneeze, laugh

or lift, this means your pelvic floor is strong enough to hold the weight of the bladder and urine for most of your activities. It is only when your activity causes a sudden strong burst of pressure that it cannot handle the strain. And thus, leaking happens. Many people with stress incontinence avoid exercising in a group (workout class or gym), jumping activities (jump rope or trampoline), or cross their legs when they sneeze. Pelvic Floor Physical Therapy is a great way to improve stress incontinence. By strengthening your core, pelvic floor muscles, and managing the pressure on your pelvic floor, stress incontinence can become a thing of the past.

Urge Incontinence:

When you have to go, you HAVE TO GO RIGHT NOW! You can be going about your day and all of a sudden, you realize you have to urinate. You get a sudden, intense urge to get to the bathroom followed by an involuntary loss of urine. That's why we call it 'urge' incontinence. You may need to urinate often, including throughout the night. Urge incontinence may be caused by a minor condition, such as infection, weakness, or a more severe condition such as a neurological disorder or diabetes. Urge incontinence is very treatable with exercise and Pelvic Floor Physical Therapy.

Overflow Incontinence:

You experience frequent or constant dribbling of urine due to a bladder that doesn't empty completely. It is like a pot that is full. When you add a little bit more water in, a little bit of water will fall out. Your bladder seems to leak just little bits of urine as it fills up, all throughout the day. Exercises to stretch and strengthen the pelvic floor can help with this.

Functional Incontinence:

For some people, a physical or mental impairment keeps you from making it to the toilet in time. For example, if you have severe arthritis, you may not be able to unbutton your pants quickly enough. You may have balance issues or pain and cannot walk to the bathroom fast enough. If there is no "urgency" associated with the feeling that you need to urinate, this type of incontinence is not so much a bladder or pelvic floor issue; the real issue is the thing preventing you from getting to the bathroom in time! In this case, we help you address the issue that is "slowing you down." Poor balance, arthritis, walking slowly, or other common causes of functional incontinence are very treatable with physical therapy.

Mixed Incontinence:

You experience more than one type of urinary incontinence. Most often, this refers to a combination of stress incontinence (leaking with coughing and sneezing) and urge incontinence, "I gotta go right now!"

Once you and your Pelvic Health Specialist determine the type of incontinence you have, your treatment plan can begin to be determined.

CHAPTER 10:
PELVIC ORGAN PROLAPSE

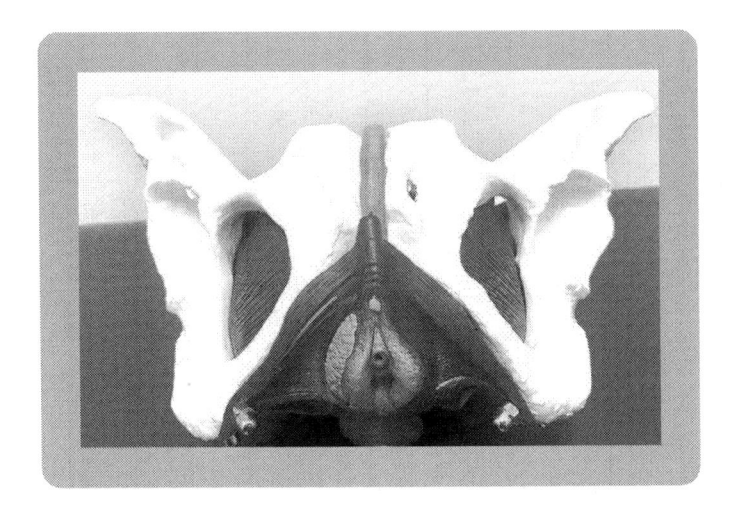

Pelvic Organ Prolapse (POP) is a Pelvic Floor Disorder that affects many women. About one-third of all women are affected by prolapse or similar conditions over their lifetime. As you recall from the earlier chapters, the pelvic floor is a group of muscles that form a kind of hammock across your pelvic opening. Typically, these muscles and the tissues surrounding them keep the pelvic organs in place. These organs include your bladder, uterus, vagina, and rectum.

What is Pelvic Organ Prolapse?

Prolapse refers to a descending or drooping of organs. Pelvic Organ Prolapse refers to the prolapse or drooping of any of the pelvic floor organs, including:

- Bladder
- Uterus
- Vagina
- Small bowel
- Rectum

Pelvic Organ Prolapse occurs when pelvic floor muscles and ligaments stretch and weaken and no longer provide enough support for the organ. As a result, the organ slips down into or protrudes out of the vagina or rectum. We will use uterine prolapse in our example below.

There Are Various Stages of Pelvic Organ Prolapse:

- Stage I – The uterus is in the upper half of the vagina
- Stage II – The uterus has descended nearly to the opening of the vagina
- Stage III – The uterus protrudes out of the vagina

- Stage IV – The uterus is entirely out of the vagina

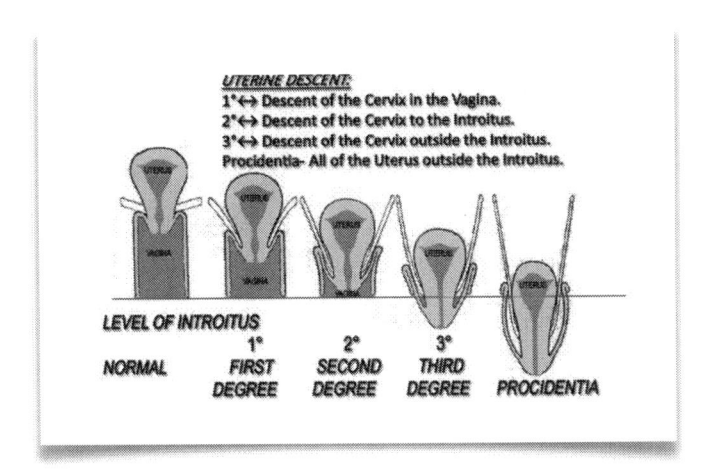

UTERINE DESCENT:
1° ↔ Descent of the Cervix in the Vagina.
2° ↔ Descent of the Cervix to the Introitus.
3° ↔ Descent of the Cervix outside the Introitus.
Procidentia- All of the Uterus outside the Introitus.

| NORMAL | 1° FIRST DEGREE | 2° SECOND DEGREE | 3° THIRD DEGREE | PROCIDENTIA |

The first picture on the left side shows the normal position of the uterus at the top of the vagina. As the stages of prolapse progress, the uterus falls farther and farther down into the vagina. Staging a POP relies on locating six defined points of the vagina. The lowest falling point is used to define the stage. If any point of the organ reaches close to the hymenal ring (the lower opening of the vagina that is felt from the outside), prolapse is usually causing your symptoms.

Stages:
- Stage I - The 1st stage or degree may have very little to no symptoms. As a result, most women do not even realize that prolapse has occurred.
- Stage II - The 2nd stage shows the uterus falling through the vagina, with at least one point reaching the base of the vagina. No portion of the uterus is visible from the outside of the body. Stage 2 is when most women can identify symptoms.
- Stage III - The 3rd stage is when the uterus protrudes outside the body. It can be seen or felt from the outside.
- Stage IV - The 4th stage is the most extreme prolapse stage. In stage 4, the organ has pushed through the vaginal wall and may be entirely outside the body.

Symptoms of Pelvic Organ Prolapse:

Mild Pelvic Organ Prolapse generally doesn't cause signs or symptoms. As Pelvic Organ Prolapse progresses, these signs and symptoms are more commonly seen. These may include:

- A sensation of heaviness or pulling in your pelvis
- Tissue protruding from your vagina

- Urine leakage (incontinence)
- Urine retention (trouble fully emptying your bladder)
- Difficulty having a bowel movement or fully emptying your bowel
- Feeling as if you're sitting on a small ball or as if something is falling out of your vagina
- Sexual concerns; feeling 'looser' in your vagina

Many people report feeling better in the morning, but the symptoms worsen as the day goes on. When you wake up, your muscles are rested and less strained. However, as the day progresses, the muscles must work harder and harder, which often causes the symptoms to appear or worsen.

Causes of Pelvic Organ Prolapse:
Remember, Pelvic Organ Prolapse (POP) results from the weakening of pelvic muscles and supportive tissues. Causes of weakened pelvic muscles and tissues include:

- Pregnancy
- Complicated labor and delivery or trauma during childbirth
- Delivery of a large baby

- Being overweight or obese
- Lower estrogen level - such as after menopause
- Chronic constipation or straining with bowel movements
- Chronic cough or bronchitis
- Repeated heavy lifting
- Placing too much pressure onto the pelvic floor

Risk Factors:

Factors that can increase your risk of uterine prolapse include:

- One or more pregnancies and vaginal births
- Giving birth to a large baby
- Increasing age
- Obesity
- Prior pelvic surgery
- Chronic constipation or frequent straining during bowel movements
- Family history of weakness in connective tissue
- More common in Hispanic or white populations

- Chronic coughing

What About My Other Organs?

The pelvic floor holds up multiple organs. Although the bladder is the most common organ to prolapse, other organs can as well (ugh). If left untreated, bladder prolapse is often associated with prolapse of other pelvic organs. You might experience:

- <u>Anterior Prolapse (Cystocele)</u>: Weakness of connective tissue separating the bladder and vagina may cause the bladder to bulge into the vagina. Anterior prolapse is also called prolapsed bladder. This is the most common condition.

- <u>Posterior Vaginal Prolapse (Rectocele)</u>: Weakness of connective tissue separating the rectum and vagina may cause the rectum to bulge into the vagina. As a result, you might have difficulty having bowel movements or fully emptying your bowels.

- <u>Urethrocele</u>: A prolapse of the urethra (the tube that carries urine).

- <u>Uterine Prolapse:</u> prolapse of your uterus.

- <u>Vaginal Vault Prolapse</u>: prolapse of the vagina.

- <u>Enterocele</u>: Small bowel prolapse.

Severe uterine prolapse can displace part of the vaginal lining, causing it to protrude outside the body. Vaginal tissue that rubs against clothing can lead to vaginal sores (ulcers.) Continuous rubbing of the sores may cause them to become infected, although this happens rarely.

When to See a Doctor:

If you show signs or symptoms of Pelvic Organ Prolapse, see your doctor or Pelvic Floor Specialist to discuss your options. This condition can become serious if it is not treated. Symptoms can become bothersome and disrupt your normal activities. But, as we will talk about later, treatment is surprisingly easy! And it is never too early to start. If you know that you have Pelvic Organ Prolapse or have had it in the past, Pelvic Floor PT treatment is very effective to reduce your symptoms and prevent a recurrence.

5 Simple Steps to Reduce Your Risk of Uterine Prolapse:
- Perform pelvic floor exercises regularly. Exercises can strengthen your pelvic floor muscles — especially important after you have a baby.

- Treat and prevent constipation. Drink plenty of fluids and eat high-fiber foods, such as fruits, vegetables, beans, and whole-grain cereals.

- Avoid heavy lifting and lift correctly. When lifting, use your legs instead of your waist or back.

- Control coughing. Get treatment for a chronic cough or bronchitis to avoid repetitive strains on your pelvic floor. If you are a smoker, the sooner you can quit or reduce your smoking, the better.

- Avoid weight gain. Talk with your doctor to determine your ideal weight and get advice on weight-loss strategies if you need them.

If you have had Pelvic Organ Prolapse surgery in the past, Pelvic Floor PT is a great way to manage your pelvic floor and ensure further complications do not occur.

When talking about Pelvic Organ Prolapse, it is never too early or too late to start treatment.

CHAPTER 11:
DIASTASIS RECTI (SIX-PACK ABS)

DIASTASIS RECTI

NORMAL ABDOMEN   DIASTASIS RECTI

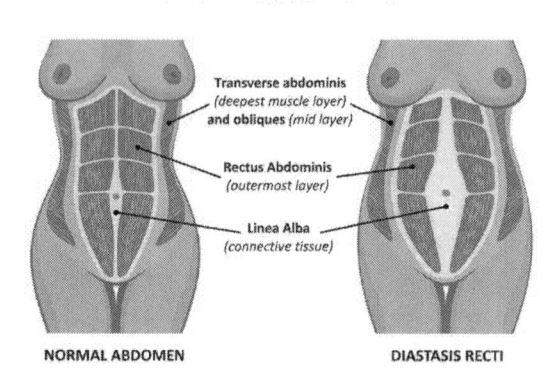

Your top layer of abdominal muscle is called your Rectus Abdominus muscle. It is commonly known as your "six-pack abs," and starts at the base of your ribs and travels down the front of your belly, attaching at your pelvis. This muscle has several tendons inside it. One thick, large tendon called the Linea Alba travels down the center of your belly, from the tip of your sternum (breastbone) to the belly button and then down to the pubic bone. This separates your six-pack abs, making three on the right and three on the left. The left side of the picture above shows a "normal" Rectus Abdominus.

When you are pregnant, there is a hormone called "relaxin" in your body, and it does exactly what it says. It 'relaxes' the tendons in your body, allowing them to expand and make room for the baby. This hormone stays in you throughout pregnancy and leaves your body about two weeks after you have your baby. If you decide to breastfeed, the relaxin will stay in your body while you nurse. However, it will stop being produced about two weeks after you finish breastfeeding.

This is good. We need our tendons to relax to make room for the baby. This hormone significantly affects your Rectus Abdominus muscle. It causes the large Linea Alba tendon to stretch and expand so your baby can fit in your belly! Unfortunately, the hormone does not distinguish which tendons are to relax (such as your pelvis and ribs) and which ones it should leave alone (such as your knees, ankles, feet, elbows, hands, etc.). This is a large component of why pregnant women have other joint issues.

So, we know the abdominal muscles need to separate - and quite a lot - to allow room for the baby. The separation in your abdominal muscles is called Diastasis Recti. "Diastasis" means separation. "Recti" refers to your ab muscles called the "rectus abdominis." Diastasis Recti is normal during your pregnancy.

Once you have your baby, Diastasis recti may get better on its own. One study showed that more than half of postpartum women had resolution of their diastasis recti by six months.

It is normal to have some space between your abdominal muscles. After all, that is how we got the look of our "six-pack abs." Normal separation is about two fingers width apart. If you want to be more precise, it should be less than 2.7 centimeters. The space between the separation should also be firm. Not hard, not squishy, but firm. It should feel like you are pushing on a trampoline. A trampoline is sturdy, but it does have some 'give' with pressure.

If you notice more than 2.7 cm separation six months or more after having your baby, OR you notice the space between your abs is more caved in or squishy, treatment by a Pelvic Floor PT is indicated to get your abdominals back into position.

IMPORTANT

If you notice Diastasis Recti after six months from having your baby, you can NOT just start doing abdominal exercises!

The Diastasis Recti is a sign that there is an imbalance in your body. If you begin doing "regular abdominal exercises" you may cause the Diastasis to worsen.

Q: I don't really care how I look. Is it still important to fix my Diastasis Recti?
A: *YES!*

Despite what our culture may make us think, your abs do so much more than make you look good in a bathing suit! One of the main functions of your abdominal muscles is to support your core. Therefore, if you have significant weakness in your abdominal muscles, you are more prone to injuring your lower back or your pelvic floor. Moms are already at high risk with all the bending, lifting, carrying, and twisting that new moms do! Therefore, we need your abdominal muscles to be strong and supportive.

Another function of your abdominal muscles is to support your digestive system. A significant amount of your digestive system sits under your abdominal muscles. If those abdominal muscles are weak and out of place, that can lead to instability in the digestive system.

Effects of Weak Abdominals on the Digestive System:
- Bloating
- Constipation
- Diarrhea
- Gas

How Do I Fix My Diastasis Recti?

Pelvic Floor Physical Therapy is awesome for this! Among other things, Pelvic Floor PT will:

- Strengthen muscles
- Improve posture
- Improve pressure management

When a Diastasis Recti does not close after pregnancy, there is a high chance that the pressure in your trunk is not being managed correctly. In other words, the gap in your belly is not closing because something continues to keep pushing it open. To effectively close the gap, we need to make sure we are moving and breathing correctly to avoid continuous straining of this area.

We will go into much more detail in the upcoming chapters of this book. Be sure to read the chapter on Pressure Management for more information!

CHAPTER 12:
HOW DO I FIX MY PELVIC FLOOR?

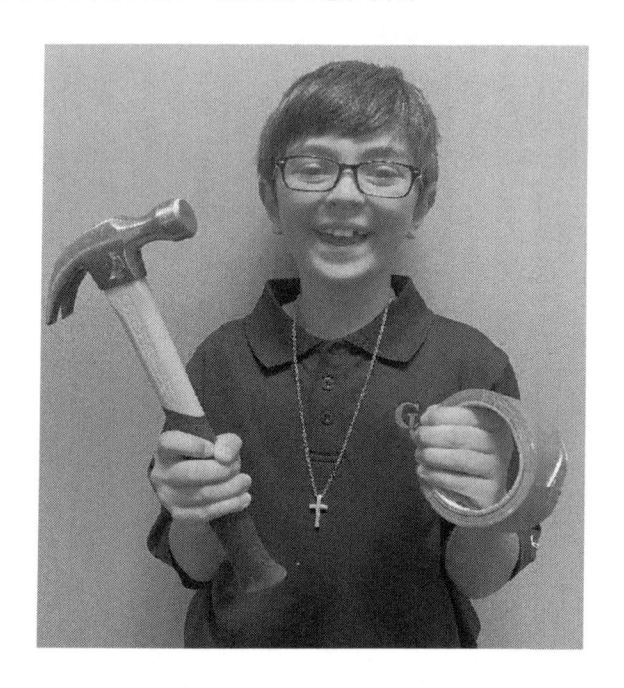

Do you think you or a loved one has pelvic floor issues? Remember, it is VERY common. As we mentioned previously, Pelvic Floor Dysfunction occurs in one out of four women under 65, and three out of four women over 65 years old. It can all seem a little overwhelming. But at the same time, it's relieving! It's relieving to know you are not alone and there is help!

So, **the BIG question is** … How do you fix Pelvic Floor Dysfunction?

Despite the picture on page 83, it is one thing we can NOT fix with duct tape! First things first, an accurate diagnosis is imperative. We need to find out *exactly* what is wrong to fix it.

Your first step in finding the answer is to schedule an evaluation by a Pelvic Floor Physical Therapist. During a complete evaluation, the Pelvic Floor Therapist can assess your symptoms, discussing any issues (leakage, constipation, pain, fullness in your groin area, pain with tampons/intercourse, etc.) you may be experiencing.

Next, the Therapist Will Look at Various Aspects Such as:

- Your past medical history
- Movement (range of motion)
- Strength
- Posture
- Tenderness of muscles
- Breathing pattern
- Pregnancy/birthing history

Surprisingly, many of these things can contribute to your Pelvic Floor Dysfunction. Weakness, pain, muscle spasms, previous surgeries, or other issues in these areas can affect your pelvic floor:

- Middle back
- Lower back
- Abdomen
- Sacroiliac joint (SI joint)
- Hips
- Thigh muscles
- Anything that affects your posture

A good Pelvic Floor PT will discuss these issues with you and assess these areas as well.

Now let's back up just a bit. Did you notice something odd in the first list of what your Pelvic Floor Physical Therapist will assess? Were any of those things surprising to you? How about breathing? Seems funny, right? Surprisingly, an improper breathing pattern is one of the MAJOR contributing factors to Pelvic Floor Dysfunction!

In the following chapters, I want to discuss "breathing patterns" in detail to see just how vitally important this is. I also want to discuss Kegel exercises. There are many misconceptions about these exercises, and we can talk about things such as:

What is a Kegel?

When should I do Kegel exercises?

How many should I do?

How long should I do the exercises?

Should I even do them at all?

I've done them before, and they didn't help one bit. Is there hope for me?

Get Ready for Our Pelvic Floor Adventure!

CHAPTER 13:
BREATHING PATTERN

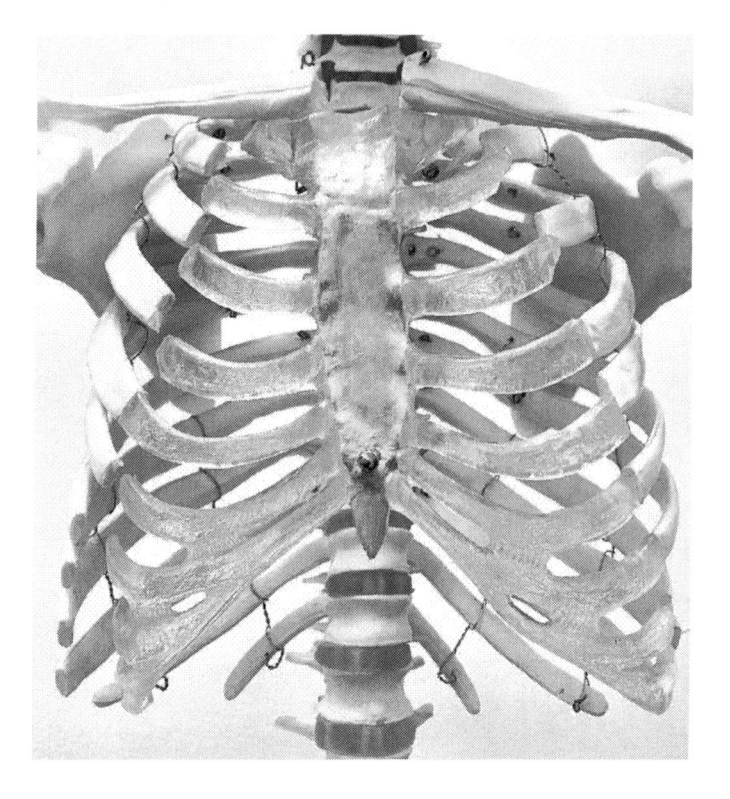

Breathing. We've done it since the moment we entered this world. It's automatic. We do it without even thinking about it. So how can we be doing it wrong?

Let's Start with the Basics:

How should good breathing look? When you inhale and take oxygen in, you should inhale deeply through your nose. This air will travel down your throat and go from the top to the base of the lungs. As you inhale deeply, the chest must expand to make room for the air.

That is where your trunk muscles come in. These are your rib muscles, diaphragm, and neck accessory muscles.

RIB MUSCLES:
Between the spaces of your rib bones are three sets of little muscles: one on the inside, one on the outside, and one in the middle. These are called innermost (inside) intercostals, internal (middle) intercostals and external (outside) intercostals. These contract and relax to allow the ribs to expand (open) the rib cage and to close the rib cage.

DIAPHRAGM:
The diaphragm is a big muscle that runs horizontally through your trunk. It is underneath your lungs and forms a "floor." When the diaphragm contracts, it pulls downward toward your belly button. When it relaxes, it rises towards the lungs and returns to its resting position.

INHALE:
When you inhale, the outside (external) rib muscles contract. These expand the rib cage and allow more room for air to come in. The diaphragm contracts and drops down towards your belly button to make the chest cavity even larger and allow more air to enter your body. This 'drops the

floor' underneath the lungs and allows for more room throughout your entire chest. As this happens and the chest cavity gets bigger, it causes a vacuum effect. This vacuum draws the air down into your body and your lungs. The farther the ribs expand and the further the diaphragm drops down, the more a vacuum is created, leading to a deeper inhalation.

EXHALE:

Have you ever thought of how the air leaves your body? How does it know that you are done with the air, and it is time for it to exit your body? That is the job of the diaphragm. As the diaphragm relaxes, it rises. The diaphragm relaxes and pulls upward, placing pressure on the lungs. In addition to the diaphragm lifting, your inside rib muscles (internal intercostals) also contract. The contraction of these muscles makes the chest cavity smaller and places pressure on the lungs. The pressure on your lungs forces the air out of your body. The more forceful the contraction, the more air is pushed out of your lungs, and the bigger your exhale becomes.

ACCESSORY MUSCLES OF THE NECK:

To help the process of lifting your chest, the front muscles of your neck gently pull up on the top ribs. Your first rib is tiny and much smaller than the other ribs. Therefore, the front muscles of the neck gently pull on your top rib to allow it to open better. These muscles are called 'accessory' because they are only helpers. They are not the primary movers of the chest.

When we are born, this is how we breathe. If you ever look at a baby, you will notice the big expansion of their chest and belly as they breathe in, followed by a strong exhale. So strong, it is easy to hear them breathe in and out, especially when they are sleeping in a quiet room.

(So precious!)

As we get older, life takes hold of us. Stress comes in. What happens to our breathing when we are stressed? We tend to breathe faster, not getting a deep inhalation or exhalation. Since we are not getting as much help from our rib muscles and diaphragm muscle on our inhale, our neck accessory muscles take over. These "helpers" end up doing a majority of the work. They can easily become overworked, causing neck, chest, and shoulder tightness.

This can be seen by taking a deep breath in front of the mirror. When you breathe in, what happens? Do your ribs open to the sides, back, and front? Or do your shoulders rise when you take a big breath? When your shoulders rise instead of your ribs moving out, this is a clue that you are not breathing with a good pattern. We call this a Shallow Breathing Pattern. Unfortunately, most adults develop this breathing pattern over time.

Have You Ever Been So Stressed or Scared That You Hyperventilate? How Does Your Breathing Look Then?
When this happens, people take shorter, quicker breaths, and there is not enough time to draw air deep into their lungs. The outer ribs do not fully contract to open the chest, and the diaphragm does not fully contract to 'drop the floor' under the ribs. Therefore, we do not get that deep cleansing breath. We do not get a deep inhalation of oxygen. And why is it essential that we get that oxygen? We need that oxygen to live! Imagine what happens when we continually do not get the oxygen we need. What happens to our energy, healing ability, and even our mood? Do you feel like this has been happening to you?

What happens to our exhale when we have a shallow breathing pattern, as in our hyperventilation example? We get a short, slight exhale. It is more of a 'heh' instead of a 'HEEEEEE' sound because we are not removing all the remaining air from our bodies. When only part of our air leaves our body, the left-over air not exhaled remains inside our lungs. Over time our lungs become filled with old, stale air. This air is taking up room, not letting any good air in, and not doing our body any good: our energy, healing ability, and even our mood suffers.

PREGNANCY:

Let's talk about those of us who have been blessed to be pregnant. When you are pregnant, where is your baby? In your uterus. As the baby grows, the uterus becomes bigger and takes up more room. It slowly pushes your organs out of the way, shifts them around, and the baby makes themselves comfortable. At first, it's not so bad. But after a while, as the baby grows, your body runs out of room. Everything is squished, cramped, moved, moved again, and smashed. Think about how those organs are now functioning with that big baby inside your body.

Your bladder gets pushed to the point that it cannot fill up as much as it used to. As a result, you do not have the space to store as much urine as you did before. So, you go to the bathroom FREQUENTLY!

Your stomach also gets pushed. You feel like you are STARVING! That your belly is EMPTY! But then, when you get food, you only eat a small portion of it. There is not enough room for the food you usually eat. So, you eat more often. These examples define the "typical pregnant woman." We even laugh about how often pregnant women go to the bathroom and eat.

But We Have Other Organs, too. What Happens to Them? Your lungs are also pushed. They do not have enough space to allow you to take a deep breath. Our ribs do not expand like before because they have been shoved and pushed to the max. So, we end up taking little breaths and breathing more frequently. Our accessory muscles in our neck start to help expand our chest as best as they can. But remember, they are not supposed to be doing all the work. They are just supposed to be helpers. With all the extra demand placed upon the neck muscles, they tend to get overworked.

Now the BIG DAY comes, we have our baby! Yay! Slowly, everything starts shifting back in place. There is more room for our bladder (yay again!), our stomach, and our lungs. Once the baby comes out, life is so relaxing. Right?! (Can you sense the sarcasm here??) All the sleepless nights, all the tending to the newborn, all the worrying, all the stress. And what happens with stress? Shallow breathing.

Women often do not fully return to their deep breathing pattern after pregnancy. Instead, the shallow breathing pattern remains. After a certain amount of time, this new pattern becomes a habit. Our bodies adapt it as our "normal pattern," continuing to breathe shallowly. This can continue for years! I have seen women in their 80s that still have that shallow breathing pattern adopted during pregnancy.

It is imperative that we return to a good breathing pattern. Our bodies need a deep inhale to pull in all the fresh new air and a strong exhale to force out the bad air. A good exhale makes room for the new air. Without this process, our bodies cannot get the air we need.

And for many of our body's functions, without oxygen, it's all downhill from there!

CHAPTER 14:
360-DEGREE BREATHING PATTERN

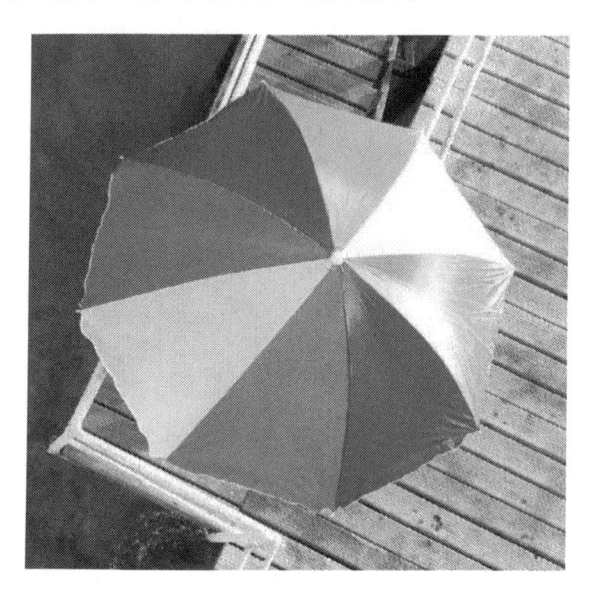

As we read in our *Breathing* chapter, we need our rib cage to expand when we breathe. We need it to get BIG to let in all that wonderful oxygen. To get the most 'bang for our buck' when we breathe, we need our rib cage to get as big as it possibly can. That means we need it to expand in all directions.

Our rib cage was wonderfully designed. Have you ever seen a rib cage on a skeleton? Where the ribs attach to the sternum or breastbone in the front is made to allow expansion.

Each rib rotates and slides where it attaches to allow maximum expansion. They also do the same where they attach in the back at the spinal column. There are three groups of super-small muscles between each rib. They move the rib from the top and the bottom, allowing each joint to expand and contract with maximum movement and strength. We are made to breathe big!

To get the maximum expansion, we want to achieve "360-degree breathing." There are three hundred sixty degrees in a circle, and for 360-degree breathing, we need our ribs to get big at every spot.

Imagine you are flying. You are up in the air and looking down on a person. You see the top of their head and the front, sides, and back of their trunk. When they take a deep breath in, you want to see expansion on ALL sides of their trunk. You would want to see the rib cage expand in the front, back, and both sides. It would be like opening an umbrella. You would see the umbrella spokes opening on all sides.

That is 360-degree breathing; the rib cage opening like an umbrella on all sides. That will maximize the air that comes into our bodies to nourish us and give life to all our vital processes. When the ribs expand during our 360-degree breathing, it gives us a more significant movement for our ribs to return to 'normal' when we exhale, resulting in a larger exhale. If we think back to

Physics Class:

$$POWER = FORCE \times DISTANCE$$

If we increase the distance (the amount of movement our ribs must travel to return to their resting position), the more POWER we will have on our exhale. This will allow us to more powerfully get rid of all the 'stale' air and release the pressure on our system.

The key to getting a big breath in is 360-Degree Breathing in our rib cage.

For some people all they need to do is to think about their breathing. Once they focus on taking that deep inhale and powerful exhale, their breathing improves by leaps and bounds. Other times there may be issues that prevent our ribcage from expanding. Of course, thinking about breathing always improves it. But for many people, there are issues preventing their ribcage from moving properly. This can be due to tightness in their upper or lower back muscles, tightness in their neck or chest, stiffness in their spine or ribs, or other issues. If this is the case, it is imperative to fix these issues to allow proper rib expansion and allow a 360-degree breathing pattern to occur. Pelvic Floor Physical Therapy is great to assess these issues and determine what issue, if any, are preventing you from your perfect 360-degree breathing pattern.

OK, now we know that we want that 360-degree breathing pattern. What happens if we do not achieve this? When we breathe improperly, this causes changes in the pressure of our abdominal cavity. However, having too much pressure in our abdominal cavity or trunk can cause several problems, none of which are pleasant, which brings us to our next chapter, *Pressure*.

CHAPTER 15:
PRESSURE

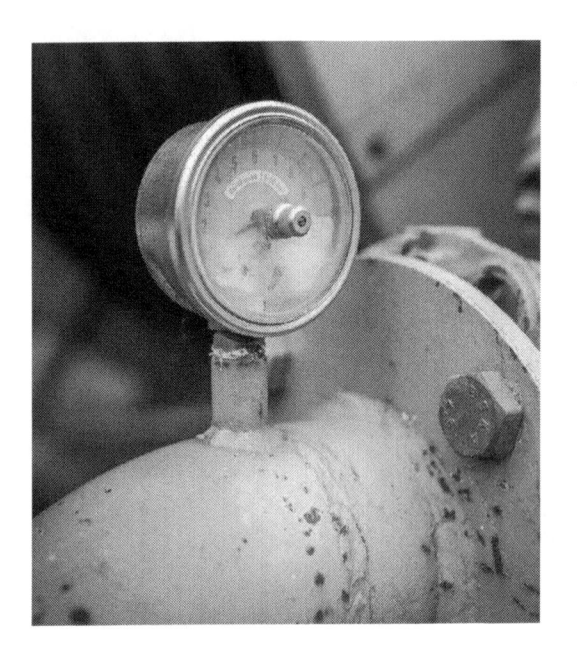

Pelvic floor issues often relate to one thing, pressure. Like many machines, your body works best with the appropriate amount of pressure. Blood pressure is a great example. We need to have the right amount of pressure in our blood vessels for them to function properly.

If there is too LITTLE pressure, the blood does not pump well through the system. The blood may pump or fall downhill into your feet without an issue; but without enough pressure, it will not have the ability to pump back uphill.

Because it does not have the ability to reach all your tissues and nourish the areas, it can cause the blood to pool in your feet. Low blood pressure also gives you other problems such as fatigue, dizziness, coldness, and weakness.

On the other hand, too MUCH pressure is bad as well. It strains our blood vessel system and overworks our hearts. It can also give us unwanted symptoms of feeling stressed, throbbing pains, headaches, and many other things.

It is important to have the correct amount of pressure in our body to work effectively and not get strained. The pressure in our trunk is the same. When we speak of the trunk, we can think of it as a box.

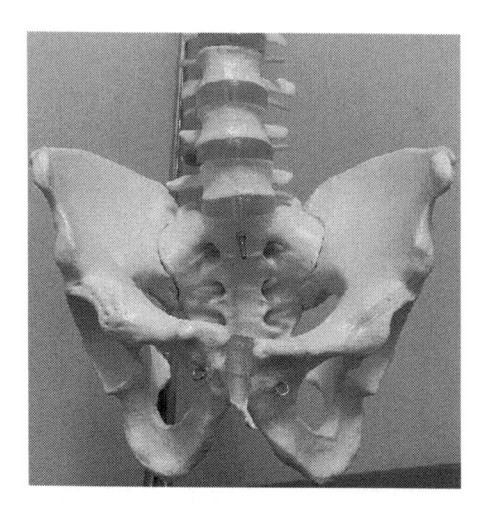

The top of our box is our diaphragm, located at the very top edge of the picture on page 100. The front is our abdominal muscles. The abdominal muscles wrap around and also form the sides of our box. The back is our lower back muscles and spinal column. And the base of our box is our pelvic floor muscles.

If we do not have enough pressure in our box, we feel weak. This is because we have no support to hold ourselves up. Without strong abdominal and back muscles, our core has no support. As a result, we have weaknesses with standing, walking, lifting, or doing things around the house. When we try to do these things, our back and abdominal muscles should carry that load. If they are not strong enough, it places that load somewhere else. Those sites are often our spinal column or pelvic floor. Too much pressure on our spinal column can lead to a bulging disc (not good). Too much pressure on our pelvic floor can strain those muscles and lead to leaking or Pelvic Organ Prolapse (also not good).

Another thing we generally do not think about is our digestive system. This system needs a certain amount of pressure to function well. If there is not enough pressure on our small and large intestines, they do not churn and digest our food properly. What do you think happens if our intestines do not push and digest our food efficiently?

What Symptoms May We Experience If Our Digestive System Lacks Pressure?

- Bloating
- Constipation
- Fatigue
- Gas
- Indigestion

Also, not good.

I don't know about you, but it is hard to do anything when my belly doesn't feel good. It's hard to focus. It just really messes up your day. So, we can all agree that we need a strong core to support our spine and pelvic floor and keep our digestive system moving properly, so we do not experience any of these symptoms.

What Happens If We Have TOO MUCH Pressure in Our Box? Let's think of a balloon. When you blow up a balloon, it has a varied amount of air you can put in it. There is a good range that you want. But it can stand a bit more pressure if you're going to blow it up more. (My son always loves big balloons. He constantly tells me, "Bigger, Mommy! Keep blowing!")

If you keep blowing and blowing and blowing up that balloon, what eventually happens? It POPS! The balloon finally must let that pressure out.

Now another question: What part of the balloon pops? Hmm, I don't really know. I guess the answer would be whatever part is strained most is where it would pop. Theoretically, it could pop at any point on that balloon. But, of course, it's hard to tell for sure on any given balloon.

What if that balloon had a weak point? Let's say before you blew up the balloon, you were stretching it out to loosen it up. One of the points may have gotten stretched just a little more than the others. If we take that balloon and over-inflate it, where would you say it will pop? It would pop where it was already overstretched, at its weakest point.

Now, Let's Go Back to Our Trunk Box:
If we put too much pressure on our trunk box, it will eventually pop, too. And where could your trunk box pop? It would pop at one of the natural weak points.

It could push pressure up the top by the diaphragm and esophagus. This could force pressure up and lead to acid reflux.

What if the pressure came out the front? It would push on your abdominal wall. The weak points in the abdominal wall are our tendons, which attach muscles to the bones. So, where are these tendons? There is a BIG one in the middle of our abdominals running right down the front of our body. It travels from the base of our sternum (breastbone) down the center of the body and attaches to the pubic bone at the top of our pelvis. This is how the tendon separates our abdominus rectus muscle and makes people look like they have six-pack abs.

1. The abdominals can separate down the center and cause Diastasis Recti, an abdominal separation common at the end of pregnancy that usually resolved in 4-6 months. However, if we continue having too much abdominal pressure after pregnancy, this Diastasis can continue.

2. The abdominals can burst at the top or the bottom of the tendon, where it attaches to the breast or pubic bone. This is commonly known as a hernia.

3. The pressure could push back into your lower back and spinal column, causing a bulging/herniated disc or other lower back pain.

4. The pressure could push down into your pelvic floor and cause leaking and possibly Pelvic Organ Prolapse.

Now, Remember That Balloon That We Stretched Out Before We Overinflated It?

If you ALREADY have weakness in any of these areas, this can be where the pressure "POPS" on you. So, if you know you have weak abdominal muscles, you may be more likely to get a hernia. Likewise, if you know you have a weak back, maybe you have had back issues in the past, you may be the one to get back pain. Or you could be the one to get acid reflux.

Finally, suppose you know you have a weakened pelvic floor (maybe you've birthed a baby, or maybe more than one baby, or perhaps you had an episiotomy or other labor and delivery issues). In that case, you may be more likely to experience Pelvic Floor Dysfunction, with or without Pelvic Organ Prolapse. Wow. Talk about yuck!

Let's Recap:

Too LITTLE Pressure Can Cause:

- Bloating
- Constipation
- Fatigue
- Gas
- Indigestion

Too MUCH Pressure Can Cause:

- Acid reflux
- Diastasis Recti
- Hernia
- Lower back pain
- Pelvic Floor Dysfunction
- Pelvic Organ Prolapse

Now we understand! Now we see why it is so vital to have our pressure system working well! I don't know about you, but I do NOT want ANY of those symptoms. That is why I'm so passionate about Pelvic Floor Dysfunction. There are way too many people going about their daily life with these issues, afraid to talk about them, and I want to help them.

Our next chapter will combine what we know about inhaling and exhaling, 360-degree breathing, and pressure. We will bring all this great knowledge together and see what happens when we do NOT breathe properly. Now is the time if you need to re-read any of these chapters. Then, when you are ready, let's see what (most of us) have been doing wrong and how we can fix it!

CHAPTER 16:
WHAT DOES BAD BREATHING DO?

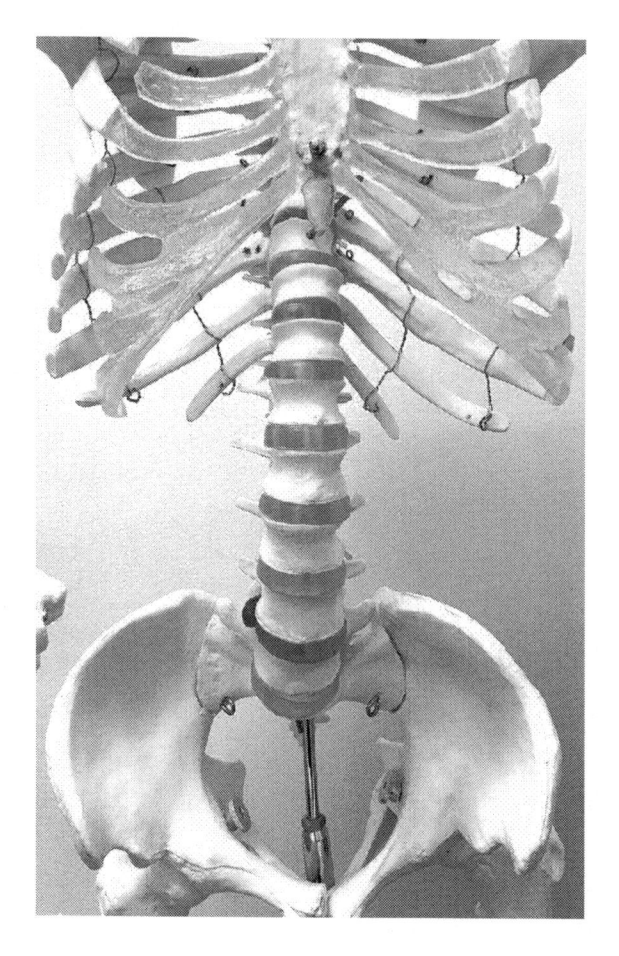

We've learned a lot! We know the mechanics of breathing, how we want to obtain 360-degree breathing, and what happens when there is too much or too little pressure on our system.

Now that we know how to breathe let's see what happens when we DON'T breathe correctly. This does get a little tricky, so if you need to re-read anything, please do.

When we do not breathe correctly, we do not get that 360-degree breathing pattern. That means something is not moving as it should; it could be the muscles in our chest, ribs, neck, or upper back. If these things are not moving correctly, it can lead to pain, stiffness, weakness, or tightness in these areas.

But there's more.

When these areas do not expand, we are not getting good air in, so we cannot give oxygen to our bodies. We really need to think of oxygen as _food for our bodies_. During improper breathing, we only inhale a small portion of the air we need to during each breath. That means that to get the right amount of air, we need to breathe more frequently. Over time, this frequent and shallow breathing pattern taxes our body. We work way harder than needed all day long. What happens when we do not get enough air or 'food?' Well, when I don't have enough food, I tend to get cranky.

But along with that, we get sluggish, tired, uncoordinated, irritable, fatigued, and things in our body just do not work right. We have low energy. We are making our bodies work way too hard all day long. And we do this because we are breathing improperly. (Am I describing anyone out there?) We need to breathe in lots and lots of oxygen to keep our bodies working right.

In addition, when we do <u>not</u> get that BIG 360-degree rib expansion on each breath, our ribs, back, neck, pelvic floor and abdominal muscles do not get adequately exercised. When we do not use muscles over time, they become tight and no longer expand. After using a poor breathing pattern for a long time, our bodies can become weak, tight or have pain in any of the areas that help us breathe. Our neck, upper back, chest, ribs, lower back, abdomen and/or pelvic floor can feel these symptoms. Basically, anything between your neck and your hips can be affected by a poor breathing pattern. Do you have tightness, weakness, or pain in any of those areas?

When we do not have a proper 360-degree breathing pattern, we lose the ability to properly regulate the pressure in our bodies.

Let's Walk Through This:
When we breathe in, we learn that our diaphragm presses down, and our ribs on all sides open up, making our trunk box bigger. When we breathe in our yummy air, it causes

more pressure to enter our bodies. There is more gas inside us, which increases the pressure inside us. When our ribs open up, not only do they allow for more air to come in, but it releases some of the pressure on the system. There is now a bigger box to accommodate the increase in pressure.

Our box remains small if our ribs do NOT move and open on all sides. There is more air in the box, but the box did not change in size. So, we have more pressure in that box. Over time, the pressure builds up and builds up. It needs to go somewhere. It places more strain on one or more sides of our box. Eventually, our 'trunk box' will POP (remember our balloon?).

And What Symptoms Can Increased Pressure in Our Trunk Box Give Us?

- Acid reflux
- Diastasis Recti
- Hernia
- Lower back pain
- Pelvic Floor Dysfunction
- Pelvic Organ Prolapse

These same symptoms can occur when we do not have 360-degree breathing because we place too much pressure on our system.

Try This Out:

Do you know anyone with acid reflux? Most of us do. It is extremely common in our society. Next time you see that person, ask them to take two deep breaths for you and watch their rib cage. I bet you that they do not have 360-degree breathing. More likely than not, when they breathe in, their shoulders go up. Their chest may come forward a little, but usually not enough. There is rarely any side rib or back rib expansion. Simply stated, their umbrella is usually not working, and they do not have 360-degree breathing.

What Other Things Can Cause Increased Pressure in Our Trunk Box?

- Exercise
- Lifting
- Straining

Now before you say, "Dr. Sara said exercise is bad for my pelvic floor." Stop. No, I am not saying that. I am saying any straining WITHOUT PROPER BREATHING is bad for your pelvic floor. Exercise is good for everyone. We just need to make sure that you are safe while doing it.

During exercise, the internal pressure in your trunk box changes. For example, when lifting a weight, the internal pressure in our trunk box increases; the internal pressure returns to normal when the weight is put down.

When I say 'lifting,' I am not only talking about lifting a weight in the gym. Yes, that is lifting. But lifting also includes bringing in groceries, picking up a laundry basket, picking up children, taking out the trash, and many other things. We lift things much more in our daily lives than we realize!

So, to maintain the proper pressure in your trunk box, you need to release pressure when you strain. This can include exercising, lifting, and even going to the bathroom (for example, when experiencing constipation).

How Do We Release This Extra Pressure?

You got it, BREATHE!

Exhaling releases that extra pressure in your trunk box. This is especially important for anyone who is already experiencing some of the symptoms we mentioned:

- Acid reflux
- Diastasis Recti

- Hernia
- Lower back pain
- Pelvic Floor Dysfunction
- Pelvic Organ Prolapse

If you are experiencing any of these symptoms, it is vital that you breathe while exercising, lifting, or straining on the toilet!

When you have these symptoms, that means there is already too much pressure in your system. Once the pressure in your balloon has popped, it is much easier to burst more often. How do we improve this? How do we take pressure off our trunk box? What happens if you just cannot get that 360 breathing pattern down?

This Is Where Pelvic Floor Physical Therapy Comes in...
Pelvic Floor Physical Therapy is essential. It is needed to retrain your system to manage this pressure effectively. Pelvic Floor PT will assess if you have too much or too little pressure, where that pressure is coming from, and how to improve it. Best yet, they will teach you how to improve it during your daily life. That way, you can get back to your life without worrying about worsening your symptoms.

Here Are Three Simple Steps You Can Take Now to Release the Pressure on Your Trunk Box:

1. Count out loud when you exercise. When you count aloud, you ensure that you exhale because you need to exhale to speak. Even if you count softly, you will be sure to improve your breathing.

2. Before you lift, exhale. When you bend down to pick up anything (laundry basket, animal food, a pan out of the oven, etc.) a split second before you lift it, exhale. Breathe out forcefully. Breathe out loudly. That makes sure that you release the pressure in your system even before the strain begins. Your pelvic floor will thank you!

3. Call a Pelvic Floor Physical Therapist for further training.

CHAPTER 17:
ALL CONVERSATIONS LEAD TO POSTURE

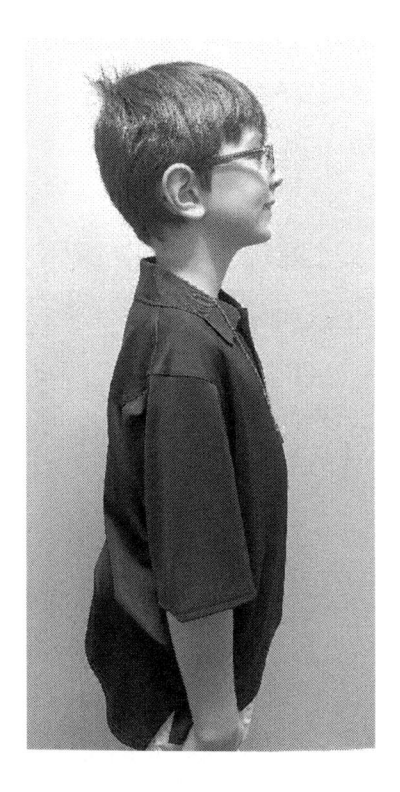

Posture. Why are we talking about posture? I thought this was a pelvic floor book! If you've ever been to physical therapy before, you know that all conversations about your body and its functions eventually lead back to posture.

Did You Know That Posture Affects Your Pelvic Floor?
Let's go back to our trunk box.

We Can Think of Our Core as a Box:

- Our rib and diaphragm muscles at the top
- Abdominal muscles in the front and on the sides
- Lower back muscles in the back
- Pelvic floor muscles at the bottom

To Have a Good Box, We Need Balance...

Our box needs to be balanced on all sides, so all sides need to be strong. If one part of our box is weak, it can collapse. We will have trouble holding things or using our box. No matter how strong one side is, our box is no longer useful if there is a weak side.

To have a sound box, we need all sides to be equal. If one side of our box is crushed, it can become shorter on that side. Then we would have a lopsided and not very useful box. It will not work right when we try to use it.

No one wants to use a crushed box. When you go to the grocery store, if you want an item - one box is crushed, and the other is intact - you pick the good box. No one wants a crushed box!

The same thing goes for our trunk box. We don't want a crushed trunk box either! If we have weaknesses in one area, our box is no longer balanced. When we try to use our core, weakness on any side will cause the box to collapse. Weakness in any part, whether your upper back, the abdominals, lower back, or the pelvic floor, will cause our core not to function correctly.

We need to be supported on all sides. If one of our areas is weak, the other side or sides will try to compensate. And it can work for a while. But slowly, the areas that are compensating are overworked. They become tight, sore, and/or painful. Eventually, one day, our body decides it simply cannot work overtime anymore. Then pain, tightness, or even part of our body 'giving way' can occur.

Now some people have a very strong body. This means your body may be able to work harder or longer to compensate for the pain. But make no mistake, everyone's body has its breaking point. Everyone has their limit. Compensation for weakness can only last for so long, no matter who you are. Then something has to give.

I also want to mention that body fat has nothing to do with core muscle imbalances. I have seen many fit people – people who work out every day, people in the military, runners, power lifters, etc. – who have muscle imbalances. An imbalance is relative. Meaning you may be very strong, but if the left side is tighter or weaker than the right, you are still not properly balanced. And you still may experience some of these symptoms.

So, all the areas of our trunk box need to be strong. And they all need to move properly.

Now let's say we sit a lot. Maybe we do a lot of computer work, reading, slouching on the couch, driving, or playing on our phone – all these activities cause us to hunch over.

This picture shows an exaggeration of slouched posture so we can see what it does to our body.

(This is the one and only time I *told* my son to slouch!)

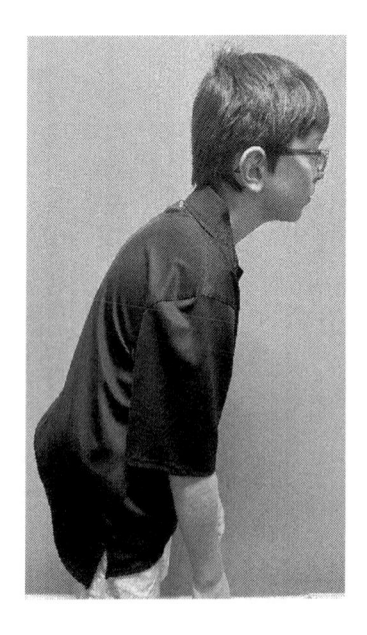

Our head comes forward, our shoulders round forward and our upper back hunches forward.

What does this do to our box? It CRUSHES it! In this picture you can see Blake's mid-section or trunk box is crushed. This crushed area of our box is now our weak point. Our muscles will eventually become weak and tight in various areas.

But a crushed trunk box does more than that. What does it do to our pressure? By crushing one area of our box, we have made it smaller. So, now we have the same amount of substance in a smaller box, increasing the pressure inside our trunk box. And what happens when our pressure increases? It pushes or "POPs" out.

What Areas Does It Push Out?

- Up onto our gastric system causing acid reflux
- Forward on our abs causing a hernia
- Forward on our lower abs causing a Diastasis Recti
- Down onto our pelvic floor causing leaking
- Down onto our pelvic floor causing Pelvic Organ Prolapse
- Back into our lower back and spine causing pain or a bulging disc

What About Below Our Box?

Can the posture below our trunk box affect it? It sure can!

Let's start from the bottom – our feet. Many people have flat feet. In fact, 70-80% of all people do not have proper arches. This flat foot posture causes our ankles to cave inward, resulting in the knees moving inward into a 'knock knee' posture. With the ankles and knees in these positions, the hips must bend forward in order to balance and stand. And where do our hips connect? To our pelvic bones. And our pelvic bones and our hip joints are where the pelvic floor muscles attach, forming the "hammock." The pelvic floor muscles are part of our trunk box. Changing the posture of our pelvic bones changes the shape of our pelvic floor muscles, and this crushes the bottom of our trunk box.

If you noticed, our legs form one chain from our feet up to our pelvic bones. Any changes in posture from our toes on up the line can cause changes in our posture further up the chain. Sometimes there are obvious changes. Other times they are very subtle. The changes in posture can cause changes in pressure all the way up to our trunk box.

In the first picture on the next page, we have a picture of a woman with pelvic floor issues standing on our ALINE Posture Assessment Device. We had her stand on the platform without shoes. Once she was correctly set up, we turned on a laser line. This line shows us where the ideal alignment of her foot, ankle, knee, and hip should be.

As you can see, she has alignment issues on her left leg (your right side when looking at the picture). The laser path goes through the center of her ankle, but it goes to the outside of her knee cap. The poor positioning of her left knee causes her hip to be out of alignment. As you can see, the laser is going to the outside of her hip joint. This was causing her hip pain with many activities.

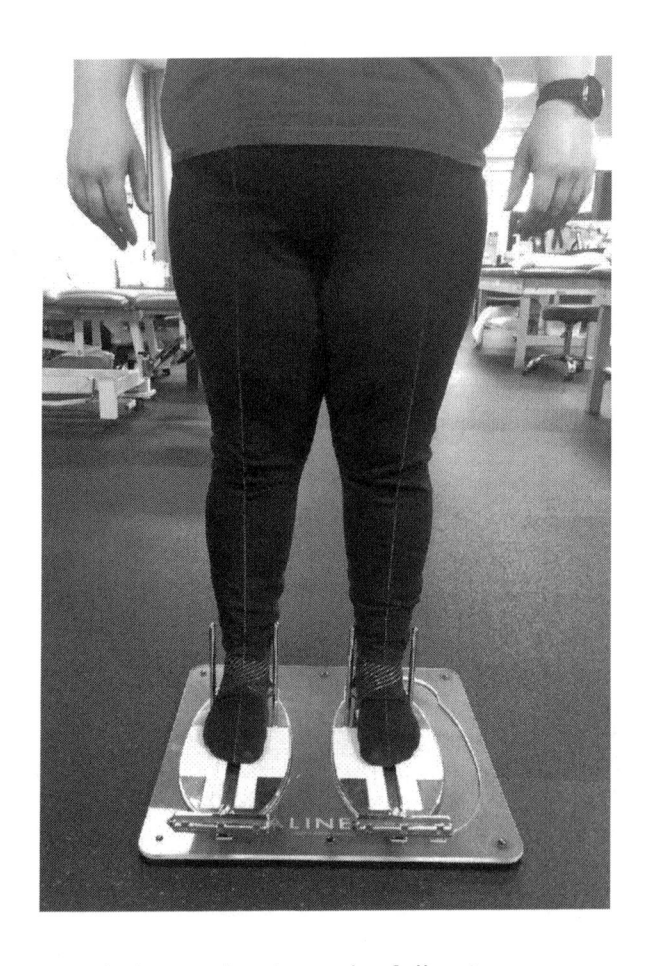

In the second picture that is on the following page, we placed orthotics inside her shoes. This allowed her foot and arch posture to improve. Once the laser was turned on the alignment of her knee and hip improved greatly. And all we did was add an orthotic into her shoe! In my clinic, we are able to further customize these inserts by heat molding them. This will fine-tune any adjustment that may still need work. What an easy fix to all the pain this was causing her!

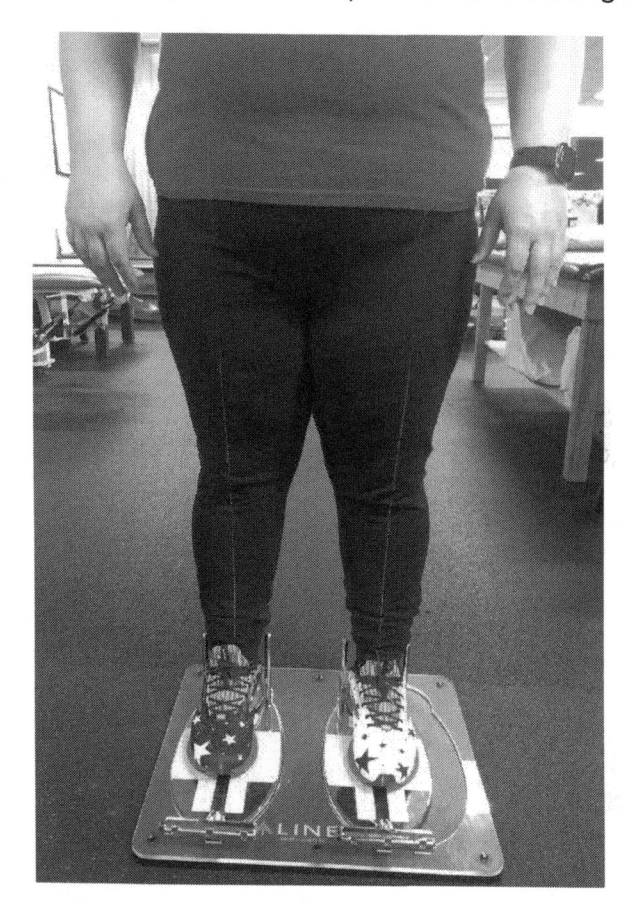

We all know from the famous kids' song: "Your heel bone's connected to your ankle bone, your ankle bone's connected to your leg bone, your leg bone's connected to your knee bone…"

Poor posture in any area can increase the pressure in our trunk. It can cause pressure to push out at any of the areas listed above and cause those symptoms. It is super important to fix your posture to help fix your pelvic floor. Even if you have been hunched over for years. If you begin to have any of those symptoms, it is time to address those issues.

> *****So, all conversations about the body DO lead to posture after all.*****

CHAPTER 18:
KEGELS

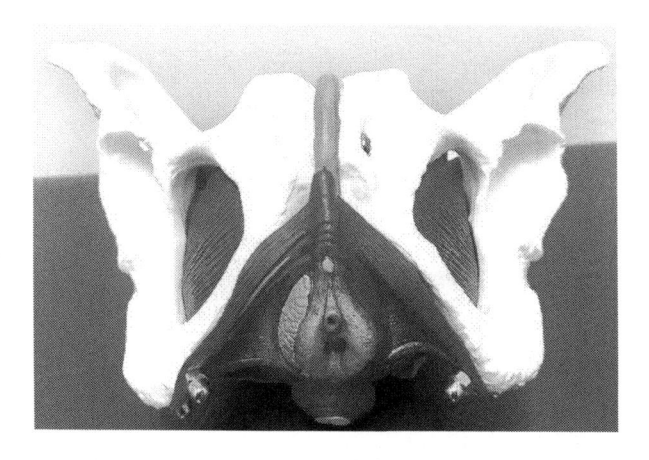

To Kegel or Not to Kegel, that Is the Question!

And what a great question it is. The answer, in short, is 'it depends.' Don't you hate when doctors say that? Let's back up and take it from the top.

First of All, what is a Kegel?

Dr. Arnold Henry Kegel was a gynecologist in the 1940s. He invented a type of exercise for women to do to prevent leaking. For this exercise, you squeeze the muscles of your pelvic floor to strengthen them. By strengthening them, you can prevent leaking and/or Pelvic Organ Prolapse. These exercises are named after him and now are commonly known as Kegels.

To do a Kegel, you simply squeeze the muscles of your pelvic floor. These can be done in several ways to train your muscles.

You Can:

- Squeeze and release quickly
- Squeeze and hold
- Slow contraction with a quick release
- Quick contraction with a slow release

Each of these patterns can train the muscles in various ways to increase your strength, endurance, and coordination.

How Do I Perform a Kegel?

This provides a challenge. Your Kegel exercises squeeze your pelvic floor muscles, which you cannot see. Even if you take your clothes off and stand naked in front of a mirror, you cannot see your pelvic floor. This makes it difficult to tell if you are doing them or performing them correctly. Therefore, there are several options to help this.

A. **The Most Well-Known and Easiest Option is Doing Your Kegels Over a Toilet.**
(Stay with me here!) First, you sit on the toilet and urinate. While urinating, you try to stop the flow of urine. So, you pee and then stop your pee. When you

stop urinating, you are contracting your pelvic floor. This exercise is a way to see if you are successfully contracting your pelvic floor muscles.

1. If you can successfully stop and start your urine flow, you are correctly contracting and releasing your pelvic floor muscles.

2. If your urine slows but does not stop, this means you may be activating your pelvic floor muscles, but the muscles are too weak to stop the flow of urine completely. Or you may be doing the Kegel improperly.

3. If you cannot stop the flow of urine, you are not activating your muscles correctly.

You should only do this to assess your ability to perform a Kegel and learn what it feels like to contract and relax your pelvic floor. Once you know this, you want to practice it off the toilet. Continual stopping and starting your urine flow every day increases your chance of a urinary tract infection, so this is ONLY for discovery purposes.

B. The Next Way to Discover If You Are Correctly Contracting Your Pelvic Floor is to Insert a Probe.

There are machines that can measure the strength and activation of your pelvic floor muscles. Specialists can insert a probe into your vaginal canal and put pads on your body. Then, they tell you to contract your pelvic floor. It will measure the strength of your contraction. It will also tell you if you are compensating with another muscle (often your abdominals or even squeezing your rear end instead of contracting your pelvic floor). You can practice squeezing and releasing while the machine is inserted to learn how to perform them correctly.

As you can imagine, this is not comfortable. Let's be honest; no one really wants a probe up there! It is also a bit embarrassing to repeatedly contract and relax your pelvic floor, with a probe and pads on, in front of a specialist staring at a computer screen. A specialist may perform this session several times until a contraction is found. If needed, sessions can continue to train and strengthen your muscles over time. Many patients do not seek treatment for their pelvic floor because they are not comfortable doing this.

C. Pelvic Floor Internal Specialist.

Another way to assess your Kegels is to have a PF specialist or OB/GYN manually insert a finger into your vaginal canal. You then contract or perform a Kegel. Not only can they sense if you are performing a Kegel, but they can assess the strength of your contraction. This is a very accurate and less costly measure. Your specialist can also give you more input than a machine can, such as if your pelvic floor muscles are tight. It can be performed once to assess for contraction and know how it feels to contract. If you have trouble contracting, you can have multiple sessions to train and strengthen over time. However, it also has that awkward, embarrassing factor.

D. Diagnostic Ultrasound.

Diagnostic ultrasound is a variation of the ultrasound you receive when pregnant. It uses sound waves to take a picture of structures in your body. It obtains a detailed, accurate picture. It can also show dynamic movements – like a video. The great thing about ultrasound is it is quick, cheap, and there is no radiation involved. With this procedure, the ultrasound probe is placed on your lower belly. (Not inside you!) You are asked to contract your pelvic floor. The ultrasound will show a real-time, dynamic, or moving picture of your pelvic floor muscles contracting and relaxing.

Diagnostic Ultrasound Can Also Visually Measure:

- The strength of your contraction
- Compensation from other muscles (the wrong muscles are working)
- The amount of movement of your pelvic floor
- Scar tissue or muscle tightness
- Coordination issues or difficulty contracting muscles correctly

Diagnostic ultrasound is rapidly becoming the favorite option for patients due to the low cost, accuracy of results, non-invasive nature, and the least embarrassing choice.

Now you know how to perform a Kegel and find out if you are doing them correctly.

The Next Question is: SHOULD I Perform Kegels?
For this question, a pelvic floor examination is crucial.

If you have weakness in your pelvic floor, Kegels will increase your strength. Proper usage of Kegel exercises can help you increase your pelvic floor's strength, endurance, and coordination. As these increase, you should improve leakage, prolapse or other symptoms.

You should NOT perform Kegels if you have a TIGHT pelvic floor.

Think about it. If your muscles are already tight and spasming, they are overworked. They are continually holding a contraction. By doing Kegels, you are asking them to continue contracting repeatedly. This is only going to aggravate the issue. As with any other muscle, the tightness needs to be worked out and relaxed before we can start strengthening. At best, Kegels will not help when you have a tight pelvic floor. Many times, it worsens the condition. It can aggravate the tightness and make the tight muscles spasm even further. Strengthening a tight pelvic floor can often cause your symptoms (leaking, etc.) to worsen. That is why we must find out if you have a tight pelvic floor before starting a Kegel program.

A pelvic floor evaluation can be a great way to discover if you have tightness in your pelvic floor. Many times, after talking and finding out what symptoms you are experiencing, an experienced Pelvic Floor Physical Therapist will be able to tell if your pelvic floor muscles are tight or not. They will also be able to refer you for a Diagnostic

Ultrasound examination to explore further any tightness, weakness, compensation, or other issues that you may be experiencing. That way, we know for sure what is going on and how to best solve your issues.

So, should you Kegel? It depends! The answer is <u>yes</u> if you only have pelvic floor weakness. The answer is <u>no</u> if you have pelvic floor tightness along with weakness. So how do we find this out? Get a Pelvic Floor Physical Therapy Evaluation. Best yet, Pelvic Floor Physical Therapy and Diagnostic Ultrasounds are covered under your health insurance!

CHAPTER 19:
PUTTING IT ALL TOGETHER

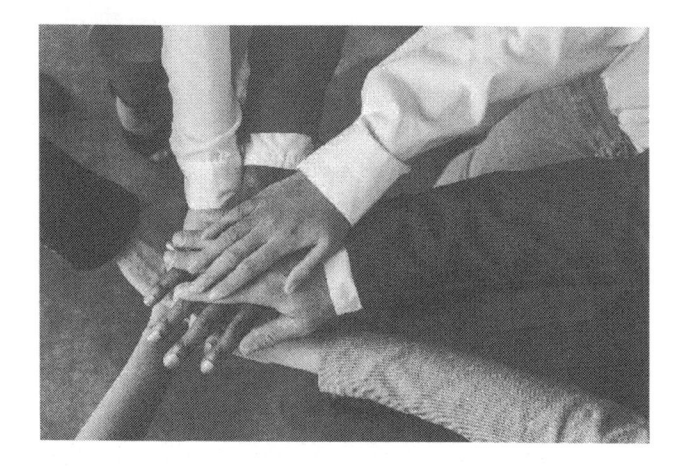

The pelvic floor is a complicated area. It serves as a connector to many places in your body.

Therefore, Issues in Any of These Areas Will Directly Affect Your Pelvic Floor:

- Abdominal muscles
- Lower back muscles
- Pelvic muscles
- Hip muscles
- Ribs
- Upper back

Furthermore, Many Areas Indirectly Affect Our Pelvic Floor:

- Breathing patterns
- Posture
- Pressure regulation

Now that we have addressed all these issues individually, we need to put them all together. Then, once we have all these areas managed and working well, we have one more thing to address: coordination and timing.

Coordination and Timing:

As with any other body area, once it is working, we need to have it working well. That means our muscles need to know when to fire or work, they need to know when to relax, and they need to understand how they need to function differently during every activity of your day. When we think of abdominal muscles, we usually think of them as one big group that functions together. In reality, each of your abdominal muscles has its own particular job. To make it even more complicated, some of these muscles, like your transabdominal muscles, have three different sections! All your abdominal muscles need to activate at different times and in the correct sequence to function properly. If this sequence is off, it will lead to issues.

Lack of Coordination and Timing in Your Abdominal Muscles Leads to:

- Instability
- Difficulty managing pressure

Let's first discuss instability. If the muscles are not strong and do not "turn on" as they should, they cannot work correctly. This can cause one area to be weak or floppy. You may feel weak when turning a certain way or doing a particular thing. Although this may cause pain, many times, there will be no pain. Some people will only experience a little 'tweak' or a 'catch' at times. Some people never have any pain with instability. They may just experience leaking of urine.

Let's say, for instance, that you have weakness in your obliques, which form the sides of your abdomen and cross over the front of your body. The obliques activate when you twist your trunk.

Let us use an example that we all do during our daily lives, vacuuming. You have to use a great deal of core strength when using a vacuum. You must push, pull, and twist to maneuver the machine. If your obliques do not fire properly when you twist, something else will have to take that pressure.

You May Compensate in Various Ways:

- You may tilt sideways instead of twisting
- You may lean back a bit and twist with only your upper back instead of the middle of your trunk
- You may step and turn your entire body instead of twisting your trunk
- You may twist at your arm and shoulder instead of twisting your trunk
- Other ways of compensation can occur

When You Do Not Use Your Oblique Muscles to Twist Your Trunk, You are Doing Two Things:

1. You are not using these muscles properly, leading to the oblique muscles getting stiff and tight from disuse. They will also become weak from not using them.

2. You are overworking other areas of your body. In our examples: other abdominal muscles, upper back muscles, hip muscles, or shoulder muscles.

You may notice these symptoms soon after your instability begins, or you may not see them for years. Often, people will realize they have pain in one area of their body without realizing that it started with compensation for pain or weakness in another area.

Difficulty Managing Pressure:

The issue that arises with poor coordination and timing of muscles is pressure management problems. In this book's breathing and posture sections, we discussed how changing the pressure in your abdomen region or your trunk box can place excessive pressure on your body. This can lead to symptoms of:

- Acid reflux
- Diastasis Recti
- Hernia
- Leaking urine and/or feces
- Lower back pain
- Pelvic pain
- Pelvic Organ Prolapse

Coordination and timing difficulties can cause these symptoms as well.

Let Us Use an Example of a Tube of Toothpaste:

To best use a tube of toothpaste, I <u>should</u> squeeze it from the bottom. Next, I would squeeze the middle section, followed lastly by squeezing the top section. That way, the toothpaste will flow through the tube and out the other end. This is an example of a well-coordinated and timed process. This is how our core would work if our coordination and timing were correct.

But let's say that our oblique muscles do not have proper coordination and timing. If my timing is off, I may fire my obliques too early. Looking at our example above, it would be like starting to squeeze one section of the toothpaste tube before I should.

I SHOULD start squeezing from the bottom of the tube, but with my timing issue, I may start squeezing from the middle. That would send some of the toothpaste out the top end as I want, but it would also send some back into the bottom of the tube. This would overload the toothpaste at the base of the tube. In this example, I have just increased the pressure in the base of the tube of toothpaste.

If we take this example and translate it back to our trunk box, we may start firing one of our abdominal muscles too early. This can cause some of our pressure to be released out the top of our trunk box into a nice exhalation. But some of the pressure would push down. As a result, the lower portion of our trunk box will be overloaded. This often leads to symptoms of Diastasis Recti, Pelvic Organ Prolapse, lower back pain, or leaking of urine and/or feces.

Now, Let's Think About What Would Happen if My Obliques Didn't Start Working When They Should, and They Fired Too Late?

In our toothpaste example, I will ideally start squeezing from the base of the tube first. Then I will squeeze the middle, followed by the top. But if my coordination and timing are off and I do not fire my muscles when I should, I could start squeezing the base of the tube. Then I would forget to squeeze the middle and only squeeze the top. What would that do?

Well, the base of the toothpaste would start moving out well. But when I did not squeeze the middle of the tube, some of the paste would get stuck there. Then when I squeeze the top of the tube, some of the paste will exit the tube as it should, but some would fall back into the middle section. So, the middle of the tube would jam up with paste from the base being pushed up along with the paste being pushed down from the top. So, I have just overloaded the middle section of my tube.

In the same manner, I can be uncoordinated with my breathing. I may bring in a deep breath of air perfectly. I get that fantastic oxygen in my body with a big, deep inhalation. But when I exhale, my coordination and timing are off. I squeeze with the lower section of my abdominal muscles and get the air moving up. But then the next section of my abdominal muscles does not fire properly. The air ends up building up in one section of my trunk box, increasing the pressure. Sooner or later, something will "POP!" And here comes that list of symptoms you know so well (acid reflux, hernia, Diastasis Recti, lower back pain, pelvic pain, leaking, and prolapse).

These examples help illustrate why not only do we need our muscles to be strong, but they need to be coordinated as well.

A Pelvic Floor Physical Therapist can help you identify if your muscles are weak, tight, coordinated, uncoordinated, and/or functioning properly together. They can also help improve your posture, breathing, and pressure management.

By Working Through These Issues, You Will Be Able to Resolve the Symptoms That Are Bothering You:

- Acid reflux
- Hernia
- Diastasis Recti
- Lower back pain
- Pelvic pain
- Leaking urine and/or feces
- Pelvic Organ Prolapse

SUPER IMPORTANT POINT

These symptoms listed above are SYMPTOMS showing that something else is wrong! When you feel these symptoms, you may suspect you have Pelvic Floor Dysfunction. You should seek treatment.

We Suspect the CAUSE of the Symptoms is a Problem in One of These Areas:

- Poor breathing pattern
- Poor posture
- Pelvic floor muscle weakness
- Pelvic floor muscle tightness

- Pelvic Organ Prolapse
- Uncoordinated muscles
- etc.

Similarly, when you have a runny nose, itchy eyes, and a headache, you suspect that you have a cold. Those are the *symptoms* of a cold. You treat the cold, not the itchy eyes.

When you experience any of the symptoms listed above, you can reasonably suspect you may have Pelvic Floor Dysfunction. Your next step should be to find a Pelvic Floor Physical Therapist for further evaluation.

CHAPTER 20:
TOP TEN COMMON PELVIC FLOOR QUESTIONS!

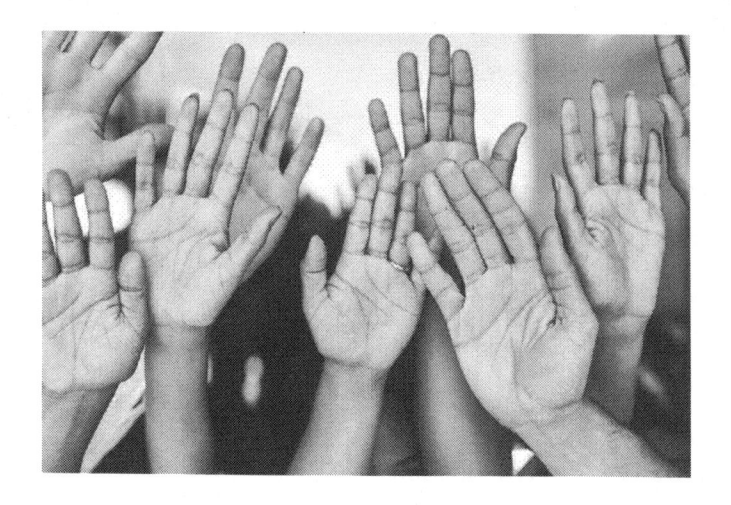

I hope you enjoyed this book as much as I enjoyed writing it! I am so passionate about helping people *Heal Your Body, Live Your Life!* – especially when we can do this WITHOUT medication, shots, or surgery!

Below are the top ten common pelvic floor questions that I receive. I hope that the answers will help you become more knowledgeable in Pelvic Floor Physical Therapy and how it can help many people get back to normal again. Remember, one out of three people under age 65 and two out of three people over age 65 suffer from these symptoms in silence! So, make sure you and your loved ones are not one of them!

1. I have heard Pelvic Floor Physical Therapy is really embarrassing. I have pelvic floor issues, but I do not want someone touching and/or massaging my genital region. Can anything be done for me?

A: This is a great question. Everyone is thinking it, but no one is saying it. I understand. No one wants someone working on them internally. The good news is you don't have to do that to get better! Pelvic Floor PT can be performed **externally for both men and women!**

By working on breathing, posture, strength, and flexibility, you would be surprised at how many internal issues can be addressed from the outside of the body! Pelvic Floor PTs are also experts on how particular massage techniques can be used on the outside of the body to correct things that are much deeper. And it's really effective!

As we all know, pain in one area of the body affects other areas of the body. So, by addressing the body as a whole, we can incorporate issues from several different areas all at once. That way, we don't get you part of the way better; we get you ALL the way better! All without touching the genitals or putting anything inside your body.

2. I have Prostate Cancer and just had surgery and/or radiation. Since the procedure, I leak urine and/or feces and cannot achieve an erection. Is there anything I can do?

A: *Yes! Yes, there is help for you!* Many men think that they have to live with urine leakage, feces leakage, or erectile dysfunction once they have prostate procedures. That is just not the case. They have significant evidence that Pelvic Floor Physical Therapy has been beneficial improving each of these issues. By increasing the blood flow to those areas, we can help the nerves regenerate. We can do specific exercises to make sure the pelvic floor muscles contract and relax correctly to improve leaking. Increasing blood flow to the penis is how erections occur and are sustained. By exercising the muscles in and around this area, we increase the blood flow. This can allow erections to be achieved and be maintained longer.

And if that wasn't good enough, Pelvic Floor PT will work on your core muscle strength at the same time. So, what have you got to lose? If you or a loved one has had prostate procedures performed, call, and speak to a Pelvic Floor Physical Therapist. Pelvic Floor PT can help with new surgeries and ones that are years old.

3. Leaking is normal as we age or after having a baby, right?
A: No! *Leaking is never normal*! It is *common* after giving birth or as we age, but never normal. Remember, leaking is a symptom. It is a symptom that there is a problem elsewhere in your body. Many times, this is caused by Pelvic Floor Dysfunction. Pelvic Floor Dysfunction is a broad term and can include problems with one or more of these issues:

- Poor breathing patterns
- Poor posture
- Pelvic floor muscle weakness
- Pelvic floor muscle tightness
- Pelvic Organ Prolapse
- Uncoordinated muscles
- Other issues

4. I have heard that Diagnostic Ultrasound can be used with the Pelvic Floor Muscles! How does this work?
A: Yes! The Diagnostic Ultrasound is a great tool to assess the pelvic floor. It is quick, inexpensive, easy, and allows static (unmoving) pictures as well as dynamic videos to be taken! That way, we can see how the pelvic floor functions at rest and with movement.

As with many conditions, pelvic floor pain usually occurs when you use specific muscles. So how amazing is it that we can not only view the pelvic floor, but we can see how it moves when you use it! Best yet, it is performed on the outside of your body. No uncomfortable or awkward probes are needed. We are blessed to have our own Certified Musculoskeletal Sonographer in my PT clinic. I can tell you firsthand how this helps quickly identify each patient's issue or issues and helps us make the best treatment plan right away. We can use ultrasound imaging instead of trial and error. That way, you get back to normal faster.

The diagnostic ultrasound can be placed on your lower belly (not inside you!) to view the muscles. Your Registered Musculoskeletal Sonographer can find all kinds of cool things like:

- Is the pelvic floor tight?
- Can you contract it?
- When you contract the pelvic floor, do you activate other muscles to compensate or activate the correct ones?
- Do the muscles move like they should when contracted?

- Can you perform a quick contraction so you can hold your bladder with a sudden impact, like jumping, coughing, or sneezing?
- Can you perform a long/sustained contraction to allow you to hold your bladder while you get to a toilet?
- It gives your Pelvic Floor Physical Therapist much more information about your condition, so you can start feeling better fast!

Since the diagnostic ultrasound is just a fraction of the cost of an MRI, they are readily approved by most insurance companies. That means you do not have to wait to receive the answers you need. No insurance? No problem! The low cost of diagnostic ultrasound makes them affordable to everyone, even without insurance.

5. I have been diagnosed with Pelvic Organ Prolapse. Is surgery my only option?

A: No! In the case of Pelvic Organ Prolapse, it is important to consider how the prolapse began. It often started with poor posture, a poor breathing pattern, inadequate pressure management, muscle weakness, muscle tightness, or incoordination. If this is the case, even if you had the best surgeon in the world, you would return to the poor habits that caused the prolapse soon after the surgery was complete. And likely, the prolapse would return.

Recent studies show that 50% of women who undergo Pelvic Organ Prolapse surgery require additional surgery.

As you can imagine, this surgery is not fun. In addition, keeping the incision clean is very difficult while on the toilet. As a result, about half of the women recommended for a second surgery decide not to get it.

Many women opt for Pelvic Floor PT first. This way, we can retrain your body's breathing pattern, pressure management, etc., to begin to take the excess pressure off the pelvic organs. By doing this alone, many patients improve to the point where surgery is not required!

Let's say, for argument's sake, you are 'that girl.' If it's going to happen, it's going to happen to you. You are always that 0.001% of the population with that horrible side effect. You are recommended for Pelvic Organ Prolapse surgery. You try Pelvic Floor PT first, and you still need surgery. During Pelvic Floor PT, we have retrained your pressure management. You now know how to do your laundry, clean your house, and take care of your grandbaby without overloading your pelvic organs with too much pressure. When you have that surgery, your body knows how to take care of itself. You no longer put excess pressure on that area. Now your surgery can successfully stay in place without additional procedures.

Of course, there are always those special instances that are so extreme they require immediate surgery. Make sure to discuss this with your surgeon.

6. I have had Pelvic Organ Prolapse surgery. It didn't help! Is there any help for me?

A: As we mentioned above, it is essential to consider how the Pelvic Organ Prolapse began. It often starts with poor posture, a poor breathing pattern, inadequate pressure management, muscle weakness, muscle tightness, or incoordination. Likely, the prolapse occurred because you experienced some of these issues. The surgery will fix the issues inside your body. It will attach things that may be loose or even completely unattached. If the surgery did not resolve your symptoms, then we know there are more factors causing you these symptoms. We need to find out what those other factors are and address them properly. Pelvic Floor PT is a great way to assess any other factors that may be contributing to your issues.

Poor posture, pressure management, incoordination, muscle weakness, muscle tightness, and poor breathing patterns are some of the frequent culprits.

The best way to ensure that you are not one of the unlucky ones who experience problems after surgery is to train your body on the correct way to manage pressure. We need to know how to manage our pressure when sitting around to relax, walk, or do more difficult things like housework, yard work, or exercise.

Pelvic Floor PT can retrain your body's breathing pattern, help build up your strength, and help you learn how to manage pressure during various situations. That way, you can get the most benefit out of your surgery.

I also want to mention that Pelvic Floor Physical Therapy works great for prolapse at any time. It can be done before surgery, shortly after surgery, or even years after your surgery! So whatever stage you are at, there is still hope!

If you recently had surgery, be sure to talk with your surgeon about the appropriate time to start.

7. I have had problems with my lower back and/or hips in the past. I am trying to get pregnant. Is there anything I can do to help me have less pain during pregnancy and childbirth?

A: This is such a great question. I hear this question from many hopeful moms concerned about how their bodies will handle pregnancy. For many people who have had pains in the past, the thought of becoming pregnant can be very scary from a physical standpoint.

Let me turn this question around: If you want to train for something, how do you go about it? PRACTICE!

Pregnancy and labor/delivery are like a race. More accurately, a marathon! You need to be strong, have good movement, and the endurance to continue for a long, long time! Pelvic Floor Physical Therapists are uniquely qualified to help you know what part of your body needs to be strong, flexible, and durable to tolerate both pregnancy and delivery. With an evaluation, we can assess those areas of the body that need to be strong and evaluate if you will be strong enough to endure a pregnancy. If not, do you think we recommend you do not have a baby??? OF COURSE NOT!!!

We help you step by step get to the point where your body is strong enough, healthy enough, and flexible enough to endure pregnancy and delivery like a champ! If you are concerned that you may not be physically able to handle motherhood (well, at least the pregnancy, labor, and delivery part), your Pelvic Floor Physical Therapist is your first stop.

8. **Help! I am pregnant and have bad pain! Is there anything that can help me while I'm still pregnant?**
A: Pregnancy is a wonderful time but does come with difficult, troubling, and painful points! One of the most aggravating things about being pregnant is no one wants to help you when you are pregnant. No one wants to take the chance that what they do will negatively affect the baby.

The good news is that you can do many NATURAL things to help Momma with her pain while not harming the baby. Exercise, stretching, and massage are great tools to help you both. In addition, Pelvic Floor Physical Therapists can help you with these pains, even during pregnancy.

There are many different types of massages. Some are safe during pregnancy, and some are not. A highly trained professional specializing in pregnancy will inform you what is safe for both you and the baby during your pregnancy.

One thing that is important to note is if your daily activities are limited by pain or other issues, physical therapy services are covered under your Health Insurance. Also, ALWAYS tell any provider or professional if you are pregnant. They may need to adjust things to make sure Momma and Baby stay safe.

9. After having a baby, my body feels "broken." Nothing works right. I really want to get back into exercising. Where should I start?

A: If you have had a baby within the past three months, your first step should be to ask your OB/GYN when you are safe to start exercise. If it is more than three months after having your baby, you can proceed to Pelvic Floor Physical Therapy. After your assessment, they will tell you what type of exercise will be most beneficial for you. Physical therapists are musculoskeletal experts. They are the best-qualified professionals to assess if you are ready for exercise and where you should begin. They will give you a program and show you where to start. Sometimes it is as simple as "You look great! You can start back at the gym. I recommend these things to start with..." Other times the PT may find something that needs a little more professional help. Either way, they are the best option to ensure you get back to 'normal' without hurting yourself.

10. It feels as if my vagina opening has "closed up." Can this be fixed?

A: Often, people have pain or discomfort in the vagina when using tampons or having sexual intercourse. It is a common misconception to feel as if the vaginal opening is 'closed-up.' Many times, the closed-up feeling is tight muscles in the pelvic floor that can become sore or painful. When any muscle is tight, it becomes shorter. The shortening of these muscles around your vaginal opening can make it feel like the hole is 'closed up.' By stretching your pelvic floor muscles, they will often loosen and stretch out to "normal length," which causes the opening to the vagina to appear to be wider. If you have had this sensation, I would highly recommend trying Pelvic Floor Physical Therapy. Pain in your vagina or during intercourse can occur for many different reasons. Be sure to mention this to your physician or OB/GYN as well. Ask them if Pelvic Floor PT may be right for you.

To wrap it up, Pelvic Floor Dysfunction is a very common issue that many people do not discuss, even with their doctors. If you have found that you or a loved one has one (or more) of the issues you have read about, ***please, please make sure to contact a Pelvic Floor Physical Therapist to help you find your next steps.***

Remember, Pelvic Floor Physical Therapy is a specialty, just like Cardiology, Neurology, or Dermatology. Not all doctors can treat you after a heart issue. In the same manner, not all physical therapists are knowledgeable about treating a pelvic floor issue. Ask if your physical therapy clinic specializes in Pelvic Floor Dysfunctions to make sure you get the best help. Feel free to contact me or your local Pelvic Floor Physical Therapy clinic for more information.

CHAPTER 21:
EXERCISES – SIMPLE WAYS TO FIX YOUR PELVIC FLOOR

With all the information you just learned about the pelvic floor, pressure, 360-degree breathing, posture and everything else… I'm sure you may be overwhelmed! Many people that I work with feel the same way. Many people tell me they knew that they had an issue, but they never realized how many issues they had! The good news is that fixing your pelvic floor issue(s) is often much easier than you expect. And most times, it can all be done without medicines, injections, or surgery.

When in doubt, breathing is a great place to start! I like to begin re-training the way we breathe. By getting the body to breathe the way it was made to breathe, we start re-forming the bad habits into good ones. As in all coordination and timing training, it is not difficult, but it does take patience. Be slow with it and give yourself a little slack. You've likely been breathing incorrectly for a long time, it may take some practice to get things back to normal.

I like to tell my patients to perform only 3-5 repetitions of each breathing exercise for each position in the morning. And to repeat only 3-5 repetitions in the afternoon or evening. No more than 3-5 repetitions to start with. Often your breathing muscles are much weaker than you think, and they will fatigue easily. In my experience many people do not necessarily feel "tired" when they practice breathing. It often feels like you started out doing them correctly, and now you can't do them right anymore. That is fatigue. Start out with only doing 3-5 repetitions twice a day. Build from there.

Will these exercises totally fix your pelvic floor and all problems associated with it?? Most likely not. As we have learned, the pelvic floor and everything that goes with it is a complex system. **This is only a starting point.** To fully get well, a full evaluation and a more specific treatment plan created for you by a Specialized Pelvic Floor Physical Therapist to address your individual issue(s) is highly recommended.

Warning: These exercises are not intended to diagnose or treat any illness or injury. It is for educational purposes only. If you choose to try any of the exercises presented here, you do so at your own risk. Please consult your physician before you start any new program. Not every exercise is safe for every person. Correct execution of all exercises is imperative to prevent injury. Please consult

your healthcare professional if you have any questions about exercise execution or if an exercise is right for you. Total Body Therapy & Wellness and Sara S. Morrison hereby disclaim any and all liability to any party for any direct, indirect, implied, punitive, special, incidental or other consequential damages arising directly or indirectly from any use of the exercises, which is provided as is, and without warranties.

90/90 360-Degree Breathing

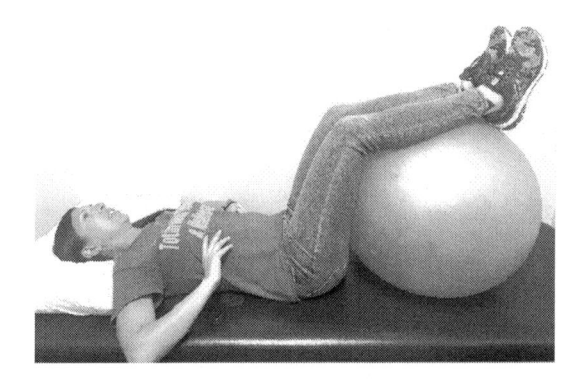

Setup
- Begin lying on your back with your legs bent at a 90-degree angle, resting on a chair or physioball. You should have your hands on the sides of your ribcage.

Movement
- Slowly take a deep breath in through your nose, expanding your ribcage to the front and sides as you inhale. Make sure you do not lift your shoulders towards your neck. Exhale from the bottom of your stomach first allowing all the air inside you to exit through your mouth. Repeat.

Tip
- Make sure not to arch your lower back. Perform slow and controlled breathing. There should not be any shoulder movement as you breath.

Side Lying 360-Degree Breathing

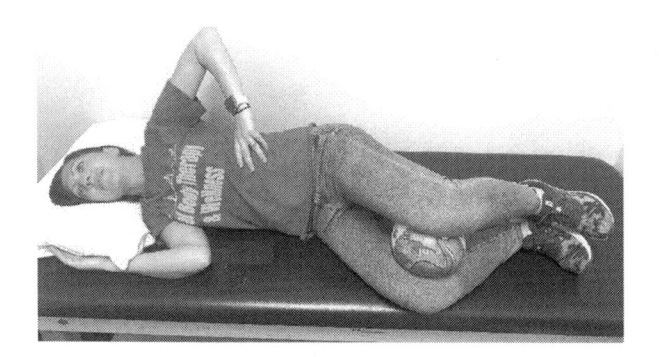

Setup
- Begin lying on your side with your knees bent and head resting on a pillow. Place a ball or pillow between your knees. Place your top hand on the side of your ribcage. Spread your fingers so your thumb is on the back side of your ribcage and your fingers are pointing towards the front.

Movement
- Inhale through your nose as you expand your ribcage to the front, side and back. Exhale through your mouth, drawing in your lower abdominals as if you are pulling your belly button toward spine.

Tip
- Make sure to focus on expanding your ribcage instead of your belly, keeping your shoulders down

away from your ears. Do not let your back arch or your hips roll forward or backward during the exercise.

Prone 360-Degree Breathing

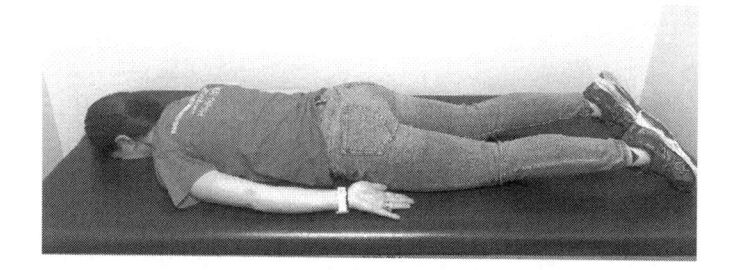

Setup
- Begin lying on your stomach with your head resting comfortably.

Movement
- Breathe in, expanding the back of your ribcage toward the ceiling. Exhale the air from the bottom, upwards.

Tip
- Make sure there is no movement in your shoulders as you breathe.

Diaphragmatic Breathing in Child's Pose with Pelvic Floor Relaxation

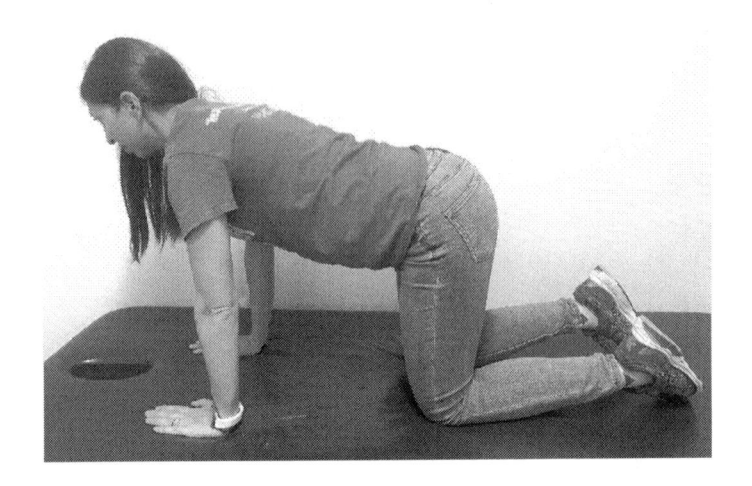

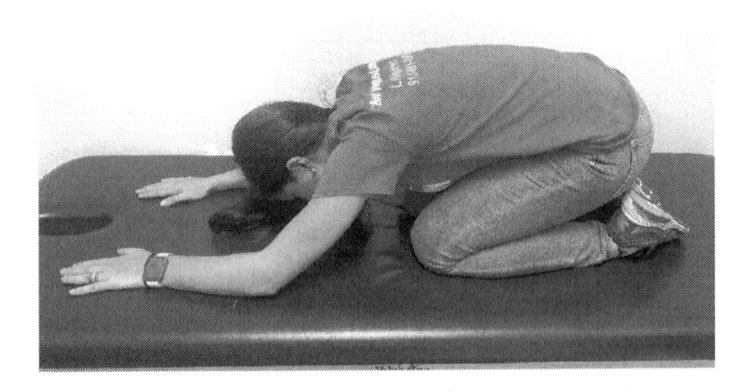

Setup
- Begin on all fours.

Movement
- Sit back on your heels, keeping your hands on the ground in front of you. Inhale, letting your chest expand to the back and sides. Envision the air travelling all the way down to your pelvic floor, allowing it to relax as you inhale. Exhale from the bottom of your belly upwards, and repeat.

Tip
- You should feel your pelvic floor muscles relax and lengthen as you inhale.

IMPORTANT POINT

These exercises are just a sample of some exercises that can help with pelvic floor issues. To achieve the best exercises for you and your specific condition, a full evaluation by a physical therapist who specializes in pelvic floor physical therapy is recommended.

Was this book helpful?
If so, please mention it to a friend or loved one. You never know which of your loved ones is one of the 66% of people suffering from
<u>Pelvic Floor Dysfunction</u>!

PATIENT TESTIMONIALS

Pelvic Floor PT works!
Don't take my word for it; ask them!

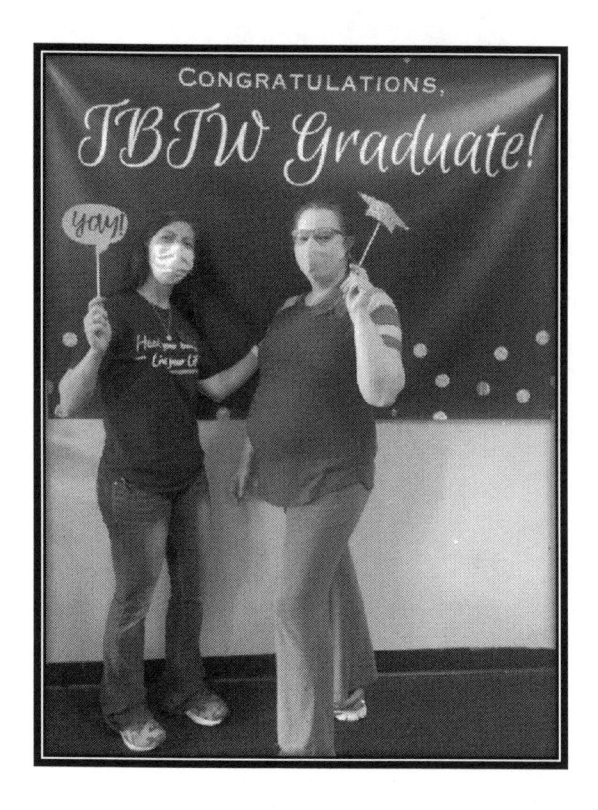

~ Anastasia Rynearson, TBTW Patient

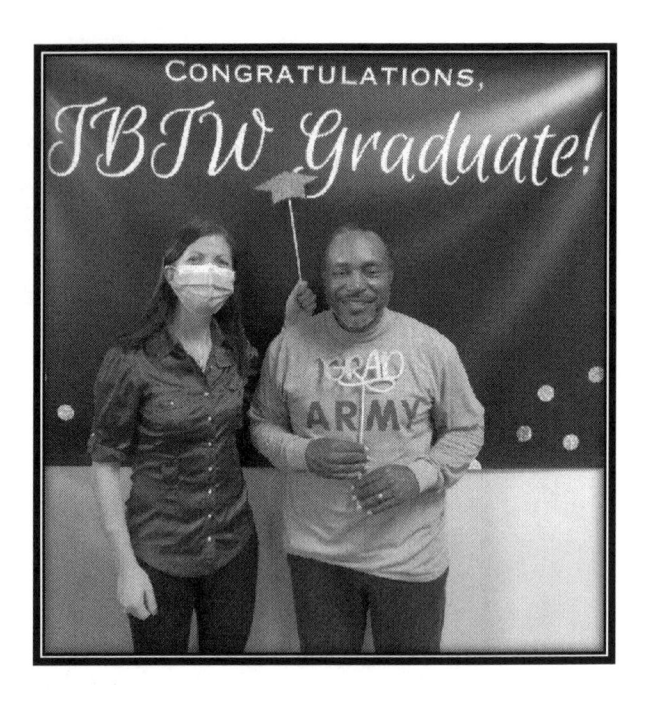

~ Palmer Mitchell, TBTW Patient

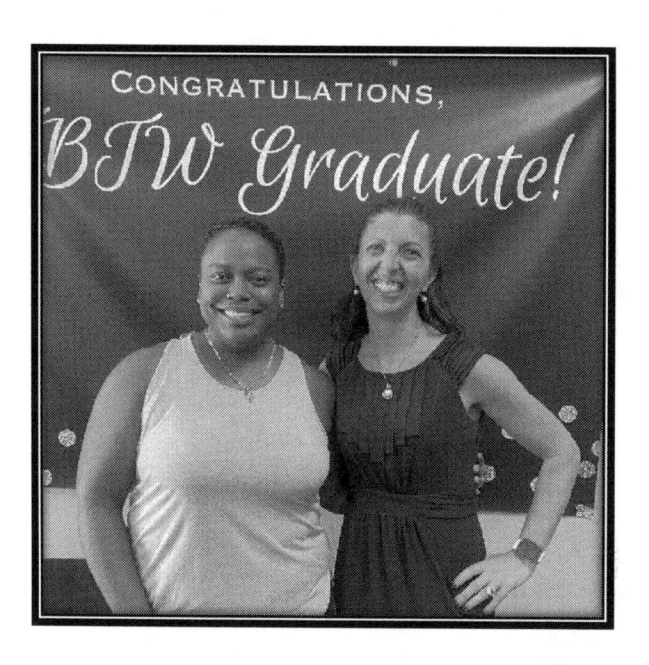

"My name is AnnLamar Johnson, and I have been practicing as a Registered Dental Hygienist for 6 years. I came to see Dr. Sara after attending a workshop that my mother had registered us for. Dr. Sara's presentation left me with a million questions; not questions due to a lack of answered questions, but questions about myself and the care I had been receiving.

At the time of Dr. Sara's presentation, I had been in physical therapy elsewhere due to injuring my shoulder in an accident. Two months in therapy and I was still out of work and my shoulder was not getting better. I just couldn't understand why, and I never questioned the care my therapist at the time was delivering as she was very good.

I scheduled an appointment for an evaluation with Dr. Sara just to get her take on things but didn't necessarily plan on switching. Dr. Sara was very thorough in her evaluation. One of the biggest differences between Dr. Sara and my therapist at the time was her specialty, experience, and vast knowledge of the pelvic floor and how it ties into the performance of the rest of the body.

When Dr. Sara started treating my pelvic floor issues which most like were a result of the accident that injured my shoulder as well, things started to improve. Prior to Dr. Sara, I never knew how important the pelvic floor health was to the function of my body as a whole. It has changed my life in so many ways.

My advice to anyone who is reading this is, it doesn't matter how old you are or your gender. Pelvic floor issues are not always caused by aging. I am only 34 years old and the same therapy my mother does for her pelvic floor issues helped me as well."

~ AnnLamar Johnson, TBTW Patient

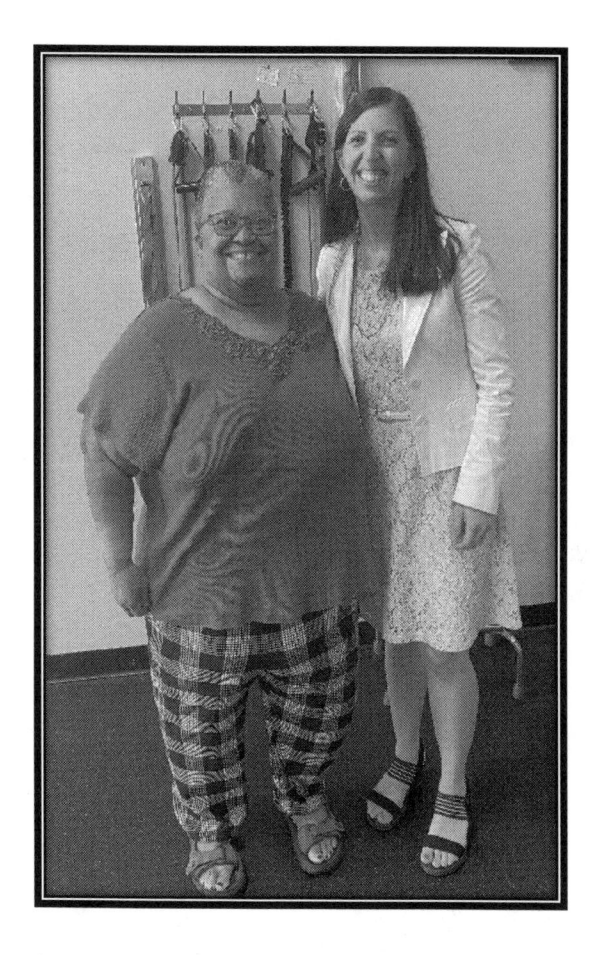

"The last three months I have been working on improving my pelvic floor strength and management, as well as increasing my core strength and stability. I was having serious incontinence issues in both areas, so much so that I would not make it to the bathroom in time and would soil myself. Since coming to TBTW I have done various exercises tailored to my issues and have also received manual manipulation to unlock some of the kinks and tightness that constricted me. I also have done home exercises recommended in tangent with 2 times a week therapy at TBTW. As a result, I am able to stand upright without falling for longer periods and have had fewer incontinence episodes. I feel more stable and secure in managing my pelvic floor. Thank you Sara, Sharon, Elizabeth and Kristin!"

~ Alvita Roberts, TBTW Patient

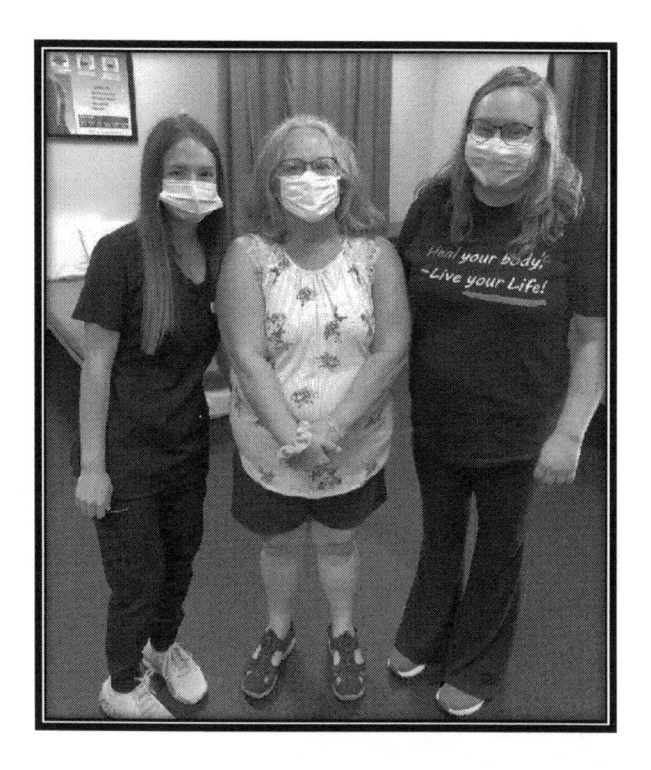

"I came to physical therapy after attending a workshop on back pain. I had pain in my lower back and right hip and at times the pain would radiate down my right leg into my foot. I was having trouble walking, doing steps, bending, and sitting. I was also having trouble with pelvic pain and incontinence. During that time, my right knee started swelling and became very painful. With many weeks of PT everything started to heal and feel better. I learned the benefits of stretching and was given many tools and suggestions to keep healing. I am now able to walk more, attend water aerobics and do everyday functions with barely any pain. PT at TBTW really saved my life. I am much more active and feeling better physically and mentally. I am stronger every day. Everyone at TBTW is very professional and caring and want you to live PAIN FREE! TBTW is a very healthy atmosphere and I really enjoyed going there."

~ Georgann Galley, TBTW Patient

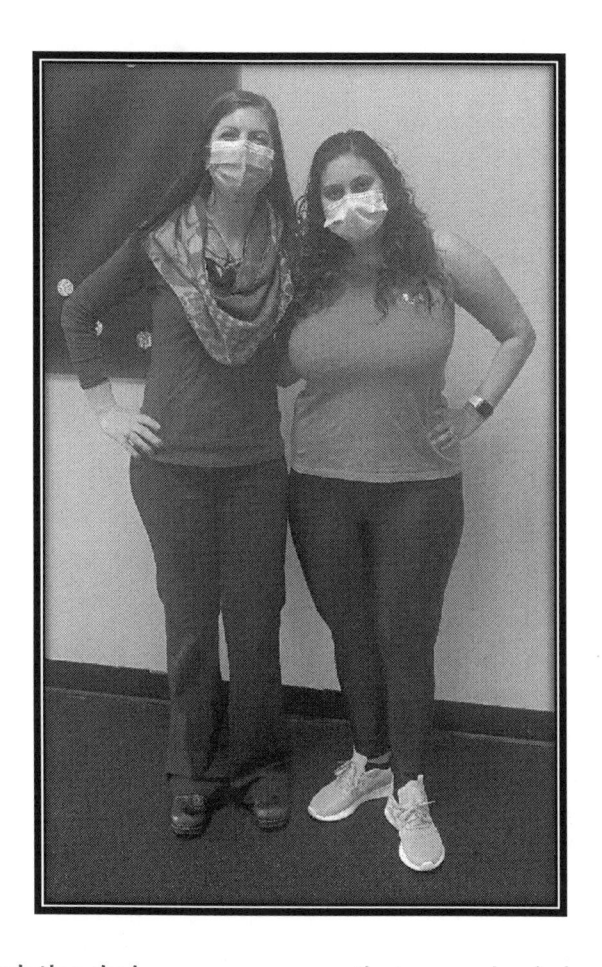

"I had sciatica during my pregnancy that caused pain in my lower back and down my leg. It hurt really bad to stand for long periods of time. I also had bladder issues that made it hard to fully empty when I urinated and made me go to the bathroom all the time! I went to PT at TBTW when I was in the last half of my pregnancy to help with the pains. After I had my son, I returned to PT to help get my body back into shape. I was having a lot of back pain when I twisted or lifted, and I was not able to work out at all.

Since I have been coming to PT, I have noticed a great improvement! My back doesn't hurt nearly as much. I can bend and lift my son pretty much as often as I need to. My abdominal separation has closed very quickly and is almost back to normal! I have been able to get back into the gym too! I am learning new exercises to help my core that are safe for me to do after having a baby. I am excited to keep working to help me get stronger, get back to all the crazy stuff I used to do in the gym and be strong enough to tolerate getting pregnant again in a year or so."

~ Suzana Abou-Zaki, TBTW Patient

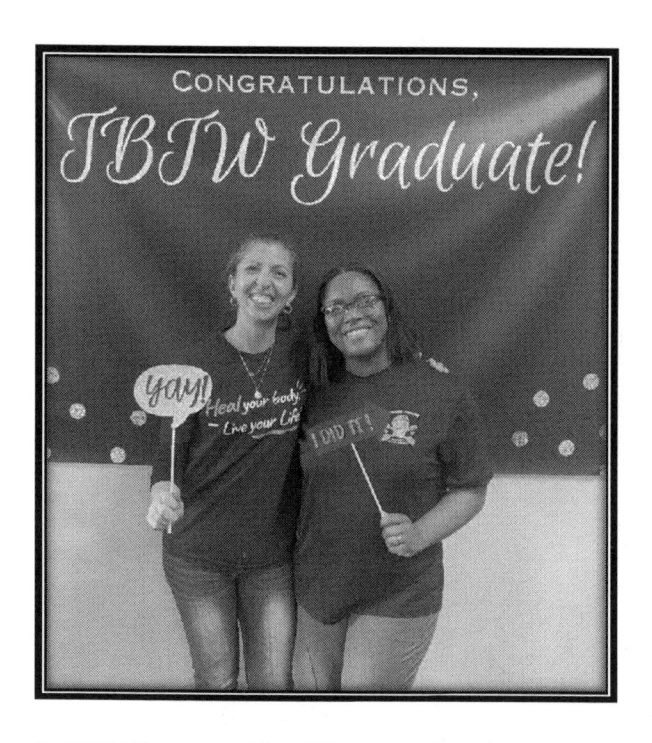

"I came to TBTW because I had Diastasis Recti. I wasn't aware that this specific condition was causing me pain almost 1 ½ years after my pregnancy. I was having stomach cramps, back pain, hip pain, and I felt so nauseated at times. I was uncomfortable doing everyday things and completing my tasks as a mom. Sara was very optimistic when I came in, even though I felt like I had waited too long to be healed. Between working out at home with the exercises she directed me to do, and the exercises and manual work Sara guided me to do in the clinic I was able to heal! I came in with a 4 cm separation at the top of my stomach and a 6 cm separation at the bottom. Now I am close to a 2 cm separation at the top and 2 cm at the bottom! I feel so much more confident in myself and my body.

My nausea has reduced, my pain has subsided and I'm so happy that I put in the work and sought help. I am grateful Sara believed in my body and didn't let me give up on myself! I will come back when I need to strengthen anything because the therapy works!"

~ Tiffany Zoeller, TBTW Patient

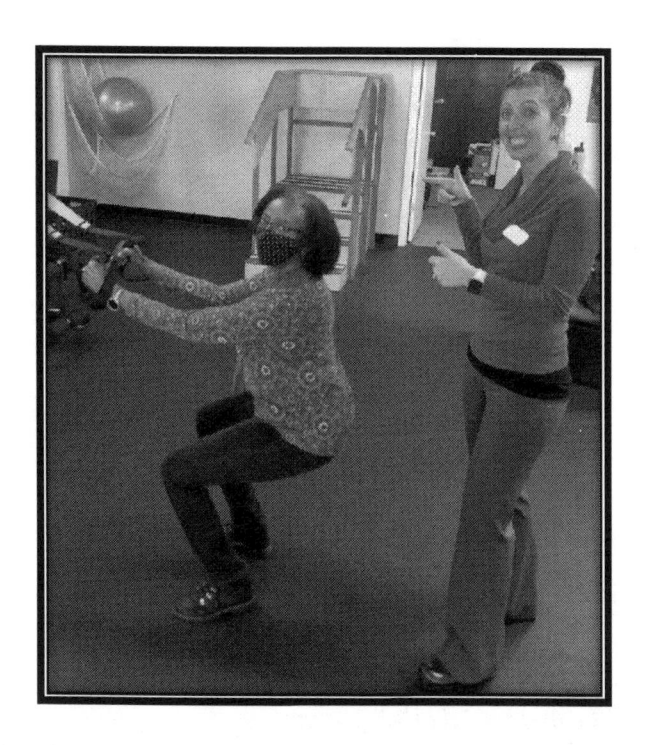

"At first, I came to Total Body Therapy & Wellness with a torn rotator cuff, and I did exercises that helped. I then realized that I could get help to strengthen my back and core since I suffer with back pain and leaking for several years. Sara and her team have helped me tremendously. I can stand longer and lift more weight without excruciating pain. I have learned how to use more of my core to do my day-to-day activities in a safe way. I do yoga classes and PT has helped me to do better in those classes. The staff is very friendly and helpful. I would highly recommend TBTW to anyone who needs to improve their quality of life. TBTW - You ROCK!"

~ Annette Johnson, TBTW Patient

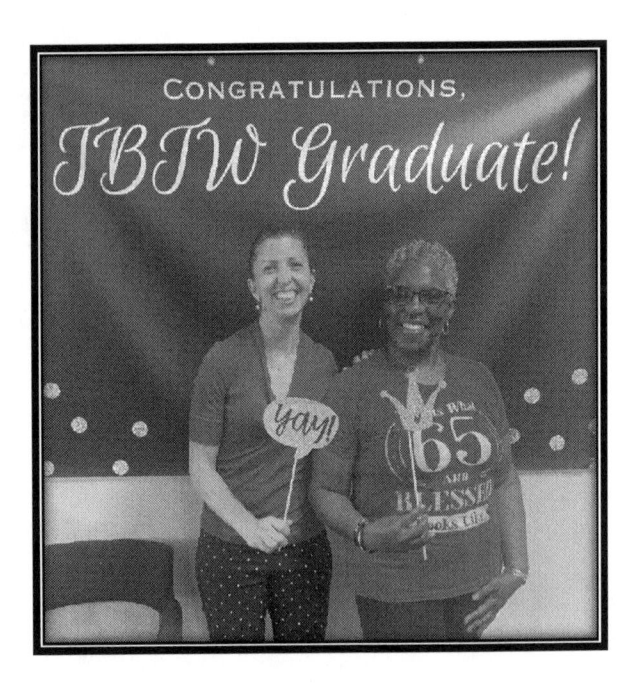

"Hello! I came to TBTW for issues with my pelvic floor. Until I attended a free Healthy Aging Workshop, I thought my issues were part of the "getting older" life. I was having issues with not being able to walk or run for exercise because it felt like my bottom was falling out and it was very painful. But that's not all - I could not hold my urine. It was like my urethra could spot a bathroom a mile away and was ready to go. I always said I was going to age gracefully, but this issue was not helping me do that. Having to always know where restrooms were on trips was a must. There was a point I started wearing underpants just like my 93-year-old mom, even at night. I woke up tired a lot of mornings because I had to get up so many times. I was also having lower back pain and could not stand very long for doing things I had to do - like cooking and taking care of my mom, never thinking that what was going on with my pelvic floor could also be connected to standing, bending, and doing other activities.

When I came to TBTW and had my initial consultation with Dr. Morrison, I cried when she said, "We can help". Within a few therapy sessions the "bottom falling out" feeling was easing and as therapy continued, the pain also left! But that's not all, as therapy continued, I began to be able to control when my urine flow started – no more leaking and just outright flowing! I wake up one or two times a night to pee and sometimes not at all. I am now able to manage pain standing through the techniques learned in therapy. It is amazing and so refreshing that what I thought was part of life turned out to be something that could be corrected.

I am so glad I overcame my shame and embarrassment to "come clean" with Dr. Morrison and tell her everything. Oh, and I can do perfect squats as part of therapy. It has been so exciting sharing with Dr. Morrison and the other therapists my wins between sessions. It was also a grand moment when I stored my remaining "aging underwear" in an offsite storage unit. This therapy has changed my life and made me more confident, secure, and just HAPPY! I know there may be others going through this same thing and feeling the same way I was. I encourage you to not be ashamed and "just live with it" but to talk about it and seek help.

Today, as I graduate, I leave with a brand-new lease on life and all it has to offer. I exercise 5 or more days a week. I decide when to go to the bathroom. I know what to do when an issue of pain occurs. They tell me here that I don't act my age, and to top it off, ALL of the staff have been amazing on this journey. They have become like family to me, as they applauded my victories and cheered me on. Dr. Morrison said, "There is help" and she was right. She said, "We can help" and they did! I am living my best life! Thank you TBTW!!"

~ Brenda Sutton, TBTW Patient

REFERENCES:

1. Pelvic Floor Disorders Network. (n.d.). *What are pelvic floor disorders?* Retrieved September 3, 2019, from https://pfdnetwork.azurewebsites.net/About/PelvicFloorDisorders.aspx
2. American Urogynecologic Society. (2017). *Pelvic organ prolapse: Symptoms & types.* Retrieved September 3, 2019, from https://www.voicesforpfd.org/pelvic-organ-prolapse/symptoms-types
3. American Urogynecologic Society. (2017). *Bladder control.* Retrieved September 3, 2019, from https://www.voicesforpfd.org/bladder-control
4. Mayo Clinic. https://www.mayoclinic.org/
5. Pelvic Floor First. http://www.pelvicfloorfirst.org.au/index.php
6. University of Chicago Medicine. https://www.uchicagomedicine.org/forefront/womens-health-articles/demystifying-pelvic-organ-prolapses#:~:text=Pelvic%20organ%20prolapse%20occurs%20as,having%20some%20degree%20of%20prolapse. Accessed May 9, 2021
7. Wiley Online Library. https://onlinelibrary.wiley.com/doi/full/10.1002/nau.23740. Accessed May 9, 2021
8. Better Health. https://www.betterhealth.vic.gov.au/health/conditionsandtreatments/prolapsed-uterus. Accessed May 9, 2021.

9. Medline Plus. https://medlineplus.gov/ency/article/000013.htm#:~:text=Time%20is%20very%20important%20when,4%20to%206%20minutes%20later. Accessed May 21, 2021
10. Biology Dictionary. https://biologydictionary.net/intercostal-muscles/ Accessed May 21, 2021
11. Pelvic Floor First. https://www.pelvicfloorfirst.org.au/pages/the-pelvic-floor-and-core.html. Accessed June 15, 2021.
12. Wikipedia. https://en.wikipedia.org/wiki/Arnold_Kegel. Accessed June 21, 2021.
13. Johns Hopkins Medicine. https://www.hopkinsmedicine.org/health/treatment-tests-and-therapies/pelvic-ultrasound. Accessed June 22, 2021.
14. https://www.hopkinsmedicine.org/health/conditions-and-diseases/prostate-cancer/prostatectomy-what-to-expect-during-surgery-and-recovery. Accessed August 5, 2021.
15. https://www.mskcc.org/cancer-care/types/prostate/treatment/radical-prostatectomy/side-effects-radical-prostatectomy. Accessed August 5, 2021
16. Allingham, C. (2020). Prostate recovery map: Men's action plan (3rd ed.). Redsok. 2. Anderson, C. A., Omar, M. I., Campbell, S. E., Hunter, K. F., Cody, J. D., & Glazener, C. M. (2015).
17. Conservative management for postprostatectomy urinary incontinence. Cochrane Database of Systematic Reviews.

https://doi.org/10.1002/14651858.cd001843.pub5 3. Asavasopon, S., Rana, M., Kirages, D. J., Yani, M. S., Fisher, B. E., Hwang, D. H., Lohman, E. B., Berk, L. S., & Kutch, J. J. (2014).

18. Cortical activation associated with muscle synergies of the human male pelvic floor. The Journal of Neuroscience, 34(41), 13811–13818. https://doi.org/10.1523/jneurosci.2073-14.2014 4. Bem, S. L. (1974).
19. The measurement of psychological androgyny. Journal of Consulting and Clinical Psychology, 42(2), 155–162. https://doi.org/10.1037/h0036215 5. Bø, K., & Finckenhagen, H. B. (2001).
20. Vaginal palpation of pelvic floor muscle strength: Inter-test reproducibility and comparison between palpation and vaginal squeeze pressure. Acta Obstetricia et Gynecologica Scandinavica, 80(10), 883–887. https://doi.org/10.1034/j.1600-0412.2001.801003.x
21. Centers for Disease Control and Prevention (n.d.) Cancer data and statistics. US Department of Health and Human Services, Centers for Disease Control and Prevention, Division of Cancer Prevention and Control. https://www.cdc.gov/cancer/dcpc/data/index.htm
22. Chung, E., Ralph, D., Kagioglu, A., Garaffa, G., Shamsodini, A., Bivalacqua, T., Glina, S., Hakim, L., Sadeghi-Nejad, H., & Broderick, G. (2016).
23. Evidence-based management guidelines on Peyronie's disease. The Journal of Sexual Medicine, 13(6), 905–923. https://doi.org/10.1016/j.jsxm.2016.04.062 8. Cohen, D., Gonzalez, J., & Goldstein, I. (2016).

24. Cleaveland Clinic. https://my.clevelandclinic.org/health/diseases/14459-pelvic-floor-dysfunction Accessed May 5, 2021.

25. Voice for Pelvic Floor. https://www.voicesforpfd.org/about/what-are-pfds/. Accessed May 5, 2021.

26. Beaumont Pelvic Floor. https://www.beaumont.org/conditions/pelvic-floor-dysfunction#:~:text=The%20primary%20causes%20of%20pelvic,women%20who%20have%20given%20birth. Accessed May 5, 2021.

27. Baby Center. https://www.babycenter.com/baby/postpartum-health/diastasis-recti_10419293 Accessed August 13, 2021.

About the Author:

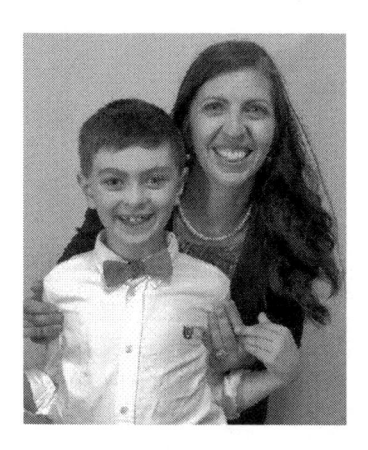

Dr. Sara S. Morrison has been a physical therapist in Harnett County since 2002. She received her Bachelor of Physical Therapy Degree from the University at Buffalo of N.Y. and her Doctorate of Physical Therapy Degree from Arcadia University. In 2008 she opened Total Body Therapy & Wellness in Lillington, NC. The goal was to provide exceptional "Big City Care" in a small-town community.

Dr. Morrison has obtained several certifications throughout her career and created several customized physical therapy programs to help heal her community. She has written five books in the *Live Your Life!* series to educate her community that natural healing is possible and effective. In addition, Dr. Morrison provides FREE books to all her patients to further their knowledge on natural healing and make the best choices for themselves.

Check out all of her books in the "Live Your Life!" series:

1. ***Heal Your Body, Live Your Life!***
   (Lower back pain and sciatica)

2. ***Improve Your Balance, Live Your Life!***
   (Balance and vertigo)

3. ***Improve Your Swelling, Live Your Life!***
   (Lymphedema, lipedema, and abnormal swelling)

4. ***Heal Your Arthritis, Live Your Life!***
   (Arthritis)

5. ***Heal Your Pelvic Floor, Live Your Life!***
   (Pelvic floor and incontinence)

When she is not working, Sara spends as much time as possible with her husband Erik, son Blake, and dogs Bella and Ellie. She enjoys running, reading, baking, sewing, watching football, and going to the beach.

SPECIAL OFFER

FREE WELLNESS CHECK-UP & DEEP TISSUE LASER CONSULTATION!

Find out how YOU can get out of pain and back to "NORMAL" faster!

Get back to the activities you enjoy today

DEEP TISSUE LASER THERAPY

Drug-Free   Surgery Free   Pain Free

LASER THERAPY RELIEVES PAIN AND INFLAMMATION ASSOCIATED WITH:

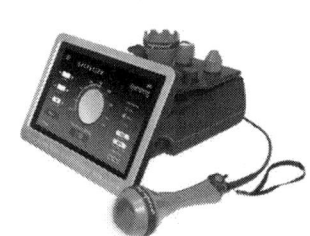

- Sprains & Strains
- Low Back Pain
- Disc Issues
- Shoulder & Knee
- Neck Pain
- Plantar Fasciitis
- Tennis Elbow
- Soft Tissue Injuries
- Carpal Tunnel
- And Much More!

Call for your FREE Consultation!
2 The Square at Lillington
Lillington, NC 27546
(910) 893-2850   www.TBTWonline.com

Made in the USA
Columbia, SC
30 June 2024